PROFESSIONAL NURSE SERIES

The Partograph and How to Assess Labour

Anna Nolte

Series editor: Nelouise Geyer

JUTA

First published 2008

The Partograph and How to Assess Labour

Disclaimer
In the writing of this book, every effort has been made to present accurate and up-to-date information from the best and most reliable sources. However, the results of nursing individuals depend on a variety of factors that are beyond the control of the authors and publishers. Therefore, neither the authors nor the publishers assume responsibility for, nor make any warranty as regards to, the outcomes achieved from the procedures described in this book.

ISBN 978 0 702 17686 9

Project management: Sarah O'Neill
Editing and proofreading: Christa Büttner-Rohwer
Cover design: Alexander Kononov
Design and typeset in 11/13 pt Berkley Oldstyle Book by Mckore Graphics Pty (Ltd)
Printed and bound in the Republic of South Africa by Mills Litho

Contents

Contents

How to use this book

This publication forms part of a series for the continuous professional development of professional nurses. The overall goal of this series is to provide an integrated approach to the topic under discussion. Each book in the series can be used by individuals or groups or as an education and training resource by nursing education institutions for learning experiences on the topic addressed.

An author who has knowledge and expertise in the particular subject has prepared each publication. It is hoped that this book will meet your learning and development needs by presenting the content in an easily accessible and user-friendly way that will facilitate learning.

Each publication addresses a specific topic in nursing, and is divided into separate chapters. The introduction includes:

- learning outcomes that you could expect to achieve after completing the course,
- the learning that is assumed to be in place, and
- key ethical and legislative considerations of which the nurse should take cognisance.

Each chapter contains:

- information and examples relating to the topic,
- learning activities with questions that allow you to apply the information in your own context,
- case study(ies) relating to the content of the chapter, and
- notes containing tips and precautions for your information, where applicable.

A separate answer guide, containing main points for consideration, is included at the back of this book.

Enjoy the learning experience!

Nelouise Geyer
Series editor
September 2007

How to use this book

Introduction

The midwife who cares for a woman during labour is responsible for recording information on the progress of labour. This progress of labour needs to be charted on a partograph, or partogram.

The partograph, or partogram, is a graphic record of progress of labour that helps caregivers detect whether labour is progressing normally or not, indicates when augmentation of labour is appropriate and assists in recognising cephalopelvic disproportion (CPD) long before labour becomes obstructed. The partograph assists nursing staff in early decision on transfer and termination of labour. It also increases the quality and regularity of all observations on the fetus and the mother during labour and aids in early recognition of problems with either. However, it is important to remember that the partograph is merely an instrument to monitor and manage labour and does not help to identify other risk factors that may have been present before labour starts.

Learning outcomes

Learners should have the appropriate knowledge and skills that enable them to use the partograph in practice to assess and interpret maternal and fetal conditions and the progress of labour to prevent and manage complications timeously, for example, maternal and fetal distress and prolonged or obstructed labour.

Specific outcomes

On completion of this course you should be able to:

- explain the principles of the partograph as a tool for prevention of fetal and maternal complications during labour
- monitor the fetal and maternal conditions, as well as the progress of labour
- record clinical observations accurately on the partograph
- interpret a recorded partograph and recognise any deviations from normal
- describe the specific midwifery actions at the appropriate time to recognise and prevent prolonged labour, and
- decide on a timely referral.

Learning assumed to be in place

The learner should have a basic knowledge of midwifery, with special reference to the assessment of a patient during labour, as well as the recognition and management of abnormalities during the first stage of labour.

Key ethical considerations

The most important **ethical consideration** in the use of specific records is honesty in recording findings.

Key legal considerations

Nurses or caregivers need to be aware that they are legally accountable for their acts and omissions. Obligations include:

- comprehensive recordings
- correct recordings
- identifying abnormalities in recordings
- interpreting findings correctly
- acting on abnormalities in recordings
- identifying warning signs of abnormalities and preventing further development of these abnormalities
- timely referral of patients in case of abnormalities.

Chapter One

The partograph

The partograph was originally designed and used by Prof. R. H. Philpott in 1972. It was later modified and simplified by the World Health Organization (WHO).

REASONS FOR USING THE PARTOGRAPH

There are various reasons why the partograph is a useful instrument to use to record progress in labour:

- **It is an assessment tool that is easy to use.** It enables nurses to see the progress of labour at a glance on one sheet of paper. Failure to progress can be recognised readily and the writing of lengthy descriptions can be avoided.
- Various studies have indicated these advantages of using the partograph: **reduction in the number of prolonged labours, labours requiring oxytocin augmentation and caesarean section** (Fahdhy and Chongsuvivatwong, 2005:301; WHO, 1994:1; Odberg Petterson *et al*, 2000:83).
- The partograph can be used by peripheral health personnel in **their referral decisions** (WHO, 1994:1), although few studies have been done on this topic (Odberg Petterson *et al*, 2000:83).
- **There is a decrease in maternal mortality and morbidity owing to obstructed labour**. Obstructed labour is an important cause of maternal morbidity and mortality. The immediate causes of maternal death resulting from obstructed labour include a ruptured uterus, complications of caesarean section and anaesthesia, postpartum haemorrhage and postpartum sepsis. In the *Third Report on Confidential Enquiries into Maternal Deaths in South Africa 2002–2004* (2006), 3 406 deaths were analysed. Table 1.1 shows the primary obstetric causes of death according to the report.

Table 1.1 Primary obstetric causes of death 2002–2004

Primary obstetric causes	%
Direct	
Hypertension	19,1
Postpartum haemorrhage	9,5
Antepartum haemorrhage	3,9
Ectopic pregnancy	1,4

>

Primary obstetric causes	**%**
Direct	
Abortion	3,5
Pregnancy-related sepsis	8,3
Anaesthesia-related	2,8
Embolism	1,9
Acute collapse	3,2
Total	**53,6**
Indirect causes	
Non-pregnancy-related infections	37,8
Pre-existing medical disease	5,6
Total	**43,4**
Unknown	3,0

(**Source**: *Third Report on Confidential Enquiries into Maternal Deaths in South Africa 2002–2004*, 2006:7.)

Recommendation 8 in this report (2006:24) concerns the correct use of the partograph: 'Correct use of the partograph should become the norm in each institution conducting births. A quality assurance programme should be implemented, using an appropriate tool.'

THE WORLD HEALTH ORGANIZATION (WHO) PARTOGRAPH

Since it first came into use, the WHO partograph has been modified and adapted by many hospitals and government authorities to suit their own needs.

There has been little research regarding different aspects of the partograph. For example, there is a lack of randomised trials determining how many hours to allow between the 'alert' and 'action' lines and whether to have two lines or only one. (Action and alert lines are discussed on page 10.) There is usually a difference of four hours between the alert and action lines. Some researchers suggest that only two hours should be allowed between alert and action. Others researchers are of the opinion that there should be one line only, suggesting that the alert and action lines should coincide (Lavender *et al*, 1998:976; Lavender *et al*, 2006:295).

There is also no research evidence that determines the most suitable intervals between assessments and the accuracy of some of the examinations, for example, the determination of cervical dilatation and the level of the fetal head.

The information in this book will be based on the principles of the WHO partograph (see Figure 1A). However, certain aspects have not been reflected on this graph, for example, deceleration of the fetal heart rate and other information obtained from vaginal examinations, for example, the position of the fetal head (see Figure 1B). The Department of Health's *Guidelines for Maternity Care in South Africa* (2002) will also be incorporated in this book.

The principles of the WHO partograph are:

- eight hours are allowed for the latent stage of labour,
- the active stage of labour commences at 3 cm cervical dilatation,
- during the active stage of labour, the woman should dilate at least at 1 cm per hour, and
- the lag time of four hours between slowing of labour and the need for intervention is unlikely to compromise the fetus or the mother and avoids unnecessary intervention.

The partograph consists of three components:

- the fetal record,
- the record of the progress of labour, and
- the maternal record.

VAGINAL EXAMINATION AND PROGRESS OF LABOUR

There is no evidence on how often cervical dilatation should be determined. Procedures vary greatly between labour wards at different clinics and hospitals and in the research literature. The number and timing of vaginal examinations should be frequent enough to permit adequate assessment of progress and detect any problems promptly, but not more frequently than necessary to accomplish this. The *Guidelines for Maternity Care in South Africa* (2002) advise that examinations should take place four-hourly during the latent stage and two-hourly during the active stage. The frequency for vaginal examinations in all the learning activities in this book is given as four-hourly in order to explain the principle. However, this interval may differ in case studies and literature.

Other features that are indicative of progress of labour are effacement and dilatation of the cervix, and descent, flexion, rotation and moulding of the fetal head, in particular. Let us look at each of these in turn.

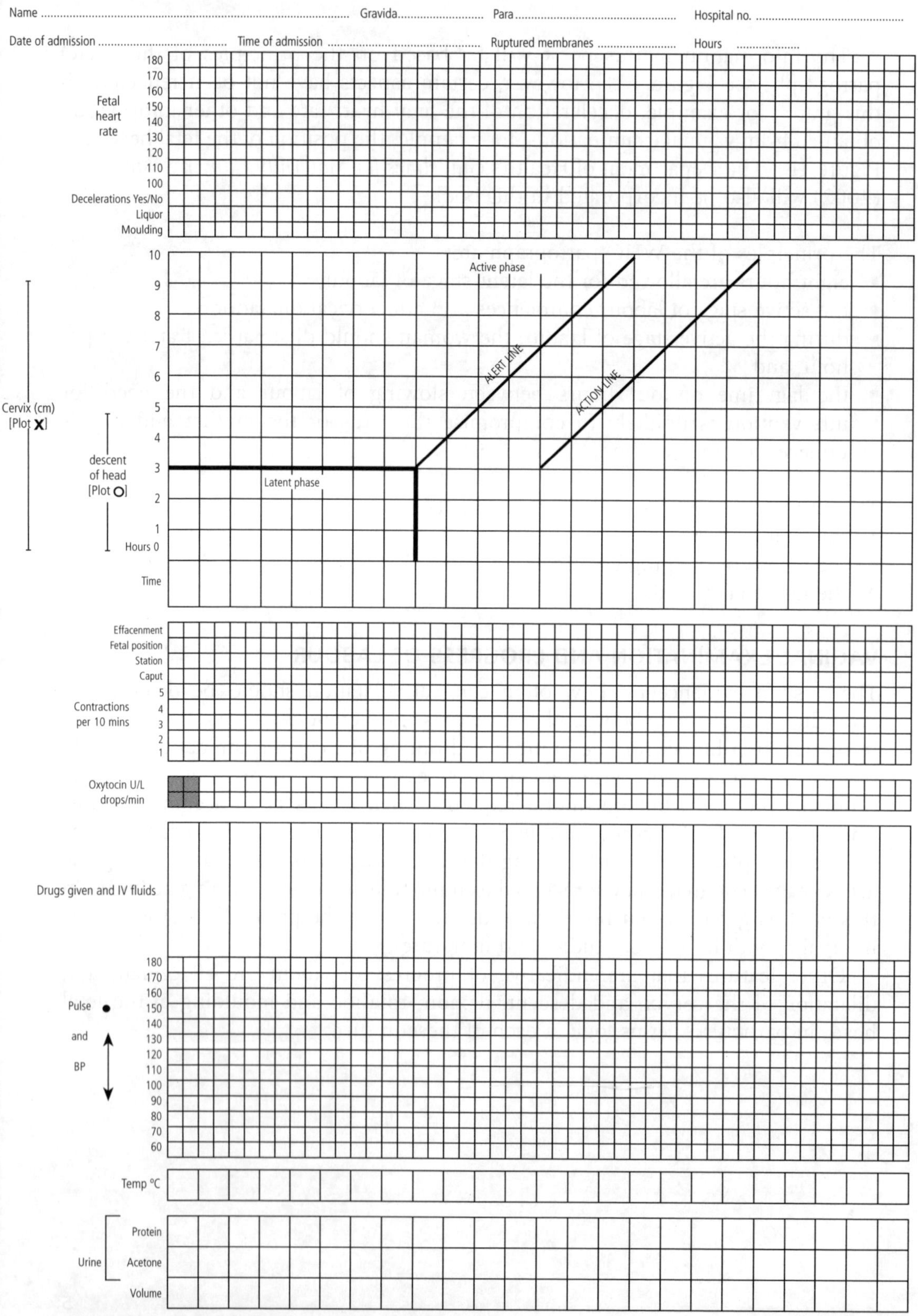

Figure 1A An example of a WHO partograph

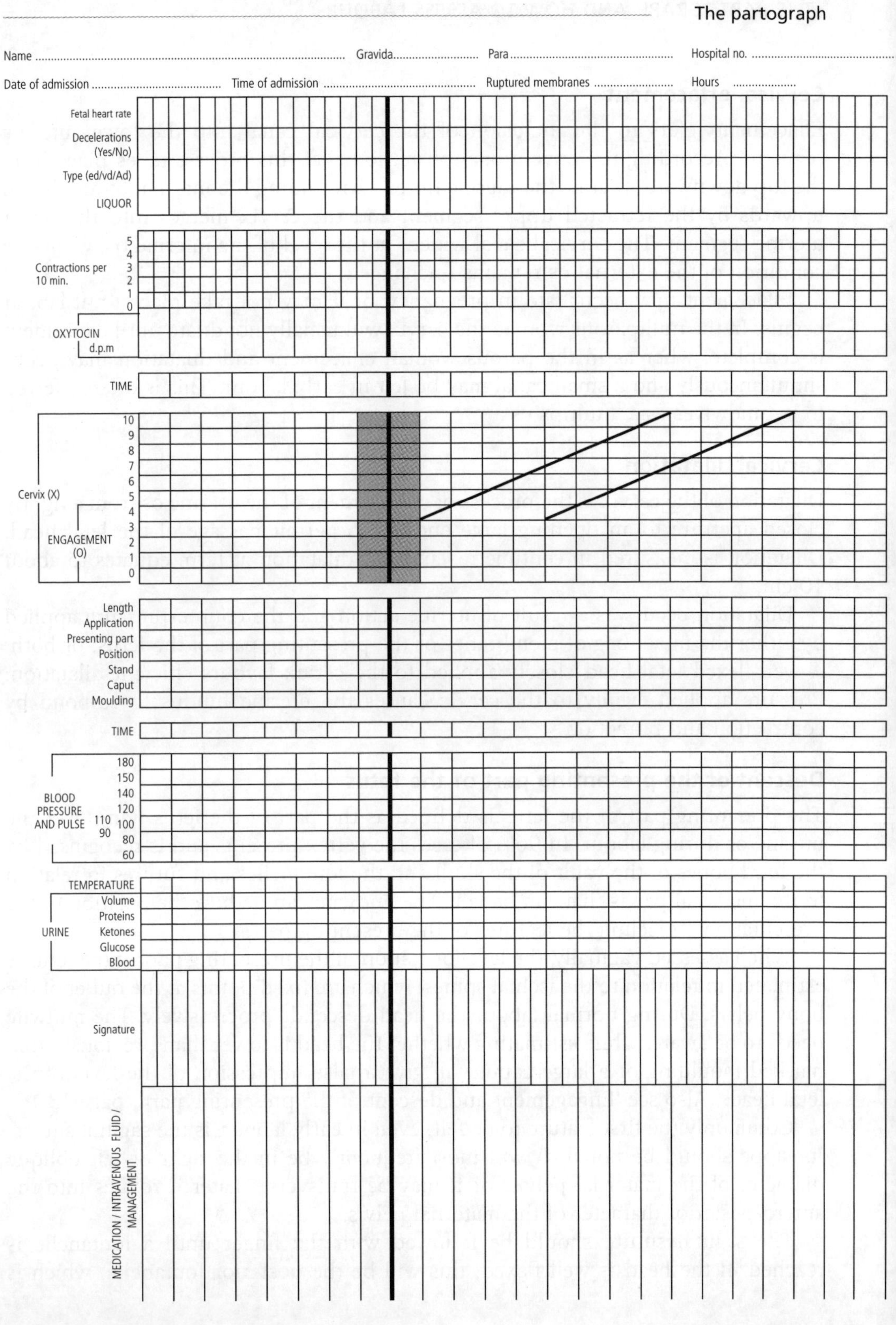

Figure 1B An example of a PEP partograph (Source: *Maternal Care Manual*, Perinatal Education Programme)

Cervical effacement

Effacement refers to the inclusion of the cervical canal into the lower uterine segment. According to conventional obstetric belief this process takes place from the top downward, that is, the muscle fibres surrounding the internal os are drawn upwards by the retracted upper segment and the cervix merges into the lower uterine segment. The cervical canal widens at the level of the internal os, while the condition of the external os remains unchanged.

Effacement may occur late in pregnancy, or it may not take place until labour begins. In the nulliparous woman the cervix will usually not dilate until effacement is complete, whereas in the parous woman effacement and dilatation may occur simultaneously and a small canal may be felt in early labour. This is often referred to by midwives as a 'multips os'.

Cervical dilatation

Dilatation of the cervix is the process of enlargement of the uterine os from a tightly closed aperture to an opening large enough to permit passage of the fetal head. Dilatation is measured in centimetres and full dilatation at term equates to about 10 cm.

Dilatation occurs as a result of uterine action and the counterpressure applied by either the intact bag of membranes or the presenting part of the fetus, or both. A well-flexed fetal head closely applied to the cervix favours efficient dilatation. Pressure applied evenly to the cervix causes the uterine fundus to respond by contraction and retraction.

Descent of the presenting part of the fetus

The presenting part of the fetus is defined as the part of the fetus lying over the uterine os during labour. In 96% of cases the vertex presents and is recognised by the hard bones of the vault of the skull and the fontanelles and sutures in relation to the maternal pelvis that can be felt. The midwife can deduce the position of the presentation by feeling the features of the presenting part.

When assessed vaginally, the level or station of the presenting part of the fetus is estimated in relation to the ischial spines, which are fixed points at the outlet of the bony pelvis. During normal labour the head descends progressively. The midwife needs to be aware, while estimating whether the head is lower than previously, that marked moulding or a large caput will give a false impression of the level of the fetal head. (Also see 'Engagement and descent of the presenting part', page 13.)

Commonly the first feature to be felt, even in early labour, is the sagittal suture. Its slope should be noted. It will most frequently be in the right or left oblique diameter of the maternal pelvis, or it may be transverse. Later it rotates into the antero-posterior diameter of the maternal pelvis.

The sagittal suture should be followed with the finger until a fontanelle is reached. If the head is well flexed, this will be the posterior fontanelle, which is recognised because it is small and triangular, with three sutures leaving it. The anterior fontanelle is diamond-shaped, covered with membrane, with four sutures leaving it. The location of the fontanelle(s) in relation to the maternal pelvis will give information about the whereabouts of the fetal occiput.

Flexion of the fetal head

In vertex presentations, progress depends partly on increased flexion. When the head is driven down on to the pelvic floor it encounters resistance: the lever principle causes the anterior part of the head to flex because there is less counterpressure. The midwife assesses flexion by the position of the sutures and fontanelles. If the head is fully flexed, the posterior fontanelle becomes almost central; if the head is deflexed, both anterior and posterior fontanelles may be palpable.

Rotation of the fetal head

Rotation is assessed by noting changes in the position of the fetus between one examination and the next. The sutures and fontanelles are palpated in order to determine position. Even if insufficient information is gained to make a definitive diagnosis, a record is made of what is felt and the findings will be evaluated with the abdominal findings at the time and compared with the findings of earlier or later vaginal examinations.

Moulding of the fetal head

This can be judged by feeling the amount of overlapping of the skull bones and can give additional information about the position of the fetus. The parietal bones override the occipital bone and the anterior parietal bone overrides the posterior.

STARTING TO USE THE PARTOGRAPH AS A RECORD OF PROGRESS OF LABOUR

Graph of cervical dilatation

This part of the graph has as its central feature **a graph of cervical dilatation against time**. It is also called the cervicogram area of the partograph. Look at the graph (Figure 2). Along the left you will see the numbers 0 to 10. Each number or square represents 1 cm cervical dilatation. The dilatation of the cervix is recorded with a cross (**X**). Along the bottom of the graph there are 24 squares. Each square represents one hour.

The cervicogram section of the partograph is divided into a latent and an active stage. The **latent stage** lasts from the onset of labour (cervical dilatation of 0 to 3 cm) until the onset of the active stage, when rapid dilatation of the cervix takes place. The latent stage is a period early in labour when uterine contractions are not yet completely organised and when the cervix is being prepared for rapid dilatation by further shortening and the process of effacement. Many caregivers regard this

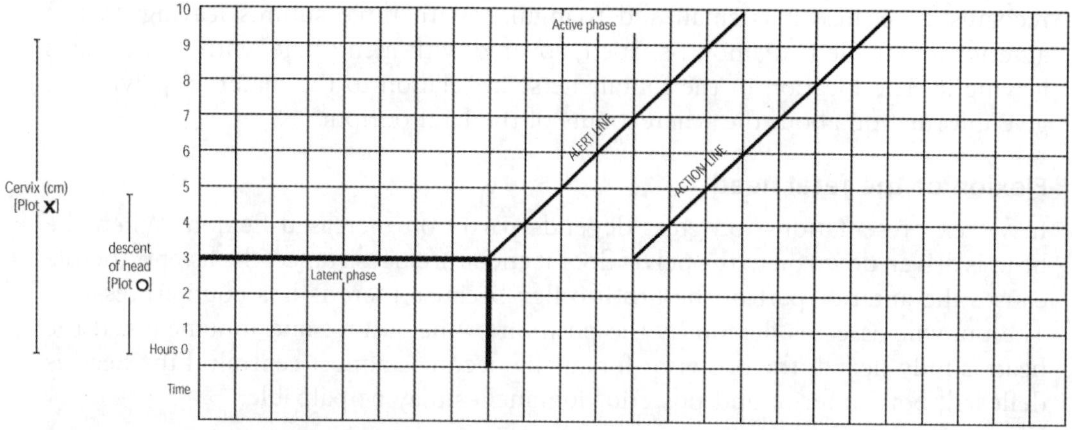

Figure 2 Labour section of the partograph (cervicogram)

as an artificial division, but the duration of the latent stage of labour should not be longer than eight hours.

The **active stage** of labour is when rapid dilatation of the cervix should be taking place (cervical dilatation from 3 to 10 cm). It is accepted that a multipara ought to dilate at 1,5 cm per hour and a primigravida at 1 cm per hour. In the normal active stage of labour a dilatation tempo of 1 cm per hour is considered normal.

In the active stage, the **alert line**, drawn from 3 cm to 10 cm dilatation, represents the rate of dilatation. Therefore if the dilatation moves to the right of the line it is slow and an indication of delay in labour. If the woman is in a peripheral hospital or clinic, she should be transferred to a hospital; if in hospital, she should be observed more frequently.

The **action line** is drawn four hours to the right of the alert line. It is suggested that if cervical dilatation crosses this line, there should be a critical assessment of the cause of delay and a decision about the appropriate management to overcome this delay should be taken. The further management of the woman in labour should be under a doctor's supervision and direction.

> **Note:** The *Guidelines for Maternity Care in South Africa* (2002) prescribe that the action line should be drawn two hours to the right of the alert line, especially in the case of community clinics that are far from hospitals or experience frequent transport delays.

It is important to note the other features that are relevant to the progress of labour, namely the **descent of the fetal head through the pelvis** and the **quality of uterine activity**.

You will now plot some graphs yourself after you have studied each example.

Example: Plotting cervical dilatation when a woman is admitted in the latent stage of labour

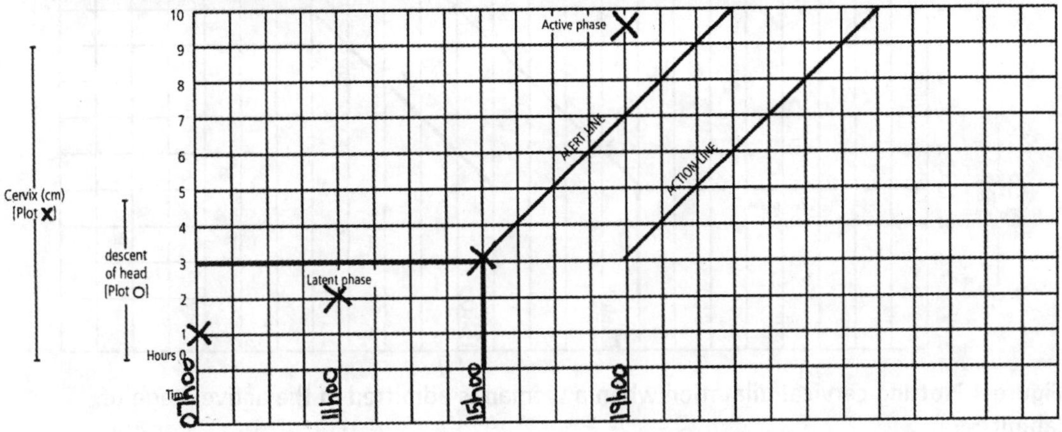

Figure 3 Plotting cervical dilatation when a woman is admitted in the latent stage of labour

Note the following on the graph above:

- The admission was at 07:00 and the cervix was 1 cm dilated.
- At 11:00 the cervix was 2 cm dilated.
- At 15:00 the cervix was 3 cm dilated.
- At 19:00 the cervix was 10 cm dilated.

Learning activity 1

Plot these data on the worksheet on page 47.

- The admission was at 14:00 and the cervix was 1 cm dilated.
- At 18:00 the cervix was 2 cm dilated.
- At 22:00 the cervix was 3 cm dilated.

Example: Plotting cervical dilatation when a woman is admitted in the active stage of labour

When a women is admitted in the active stage, the dilatation of the cervix is plotted on the alert line, at the place equal to her dilatation, with the clock time written directly under the X (of cervical dilatation) in the space for time.

Note the following on the graph (see Figure 4):

- The admission was at 09:00 and the cervix was 4 cm dilated.
- At 13:00 the cervix was 10 cm dilated.

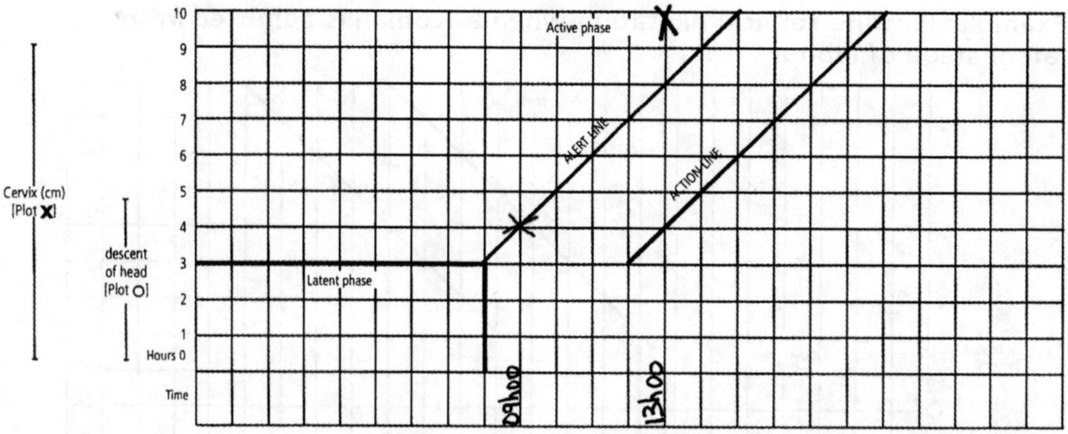

Figure 4 Plotting cervical dilatation when a woman is admitted in the active stage of labour

Learning activity 2

Now plot these data on the worksheet on page 47.

- The admission was at 12:00 and the cervix was 5 cm dilated.
- At 16:00 the cervix was 9 cm dilated.

Example: Plotting cervical dilatation when a woman is admitted in the latent stage, but proceeds to the active stage before eight hours have elapsed

When dilatation is 0 to 3 cm, plotting should take place in the latent stage of the graph. When labour goes into the active stage, plotting must be moved to the alert line by a broken line.

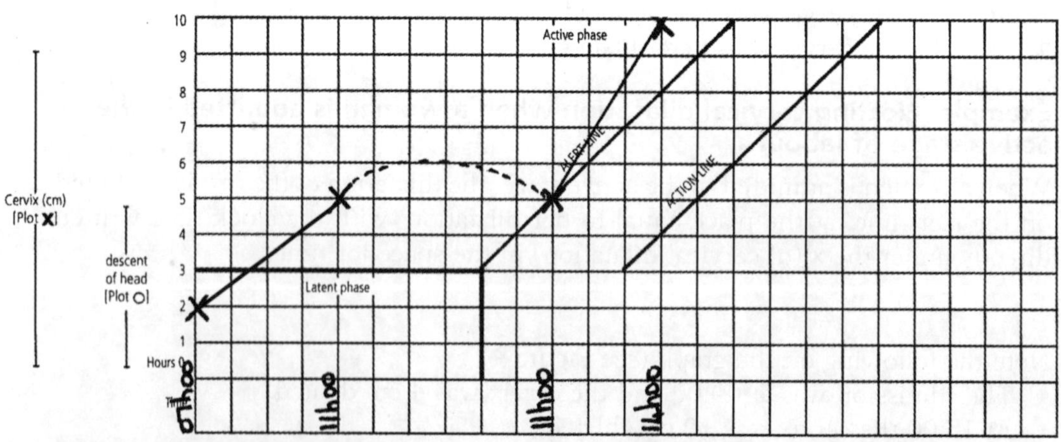

Figure 5 Plotting cervical dilatation when a woman is admitted in the latent stage, but proceeds to the active stage before eight hours have elapsed

Note the following on the graph (see Figure 5):

- The admission was at 07:00 and the cervix was 2 cm dilated.
- At 11:00 the cervix was 5 cm dilated.
- At 14:00 the cervix was 10 cm dilated.

Note: When labour is progressing well, the graph showing dilatation should not cross to the right of the alert line.

Learning activity 3

Now plot these data on the worksheet on page 48.

- The admission was at 09:00 and the cervix was 1 cm dilated.
- At 13:00 the cervix was 6 cm dilated.
- At 17:00 the cervix was 10 cm dilated.

Engagement and descent of the presenting part

Cephalic presentation

In cases of a cephalic presentation, the fetal head is engaged when the biparietal diameter passes through the plane of the pelvic inlet. In the primigravida the fetal head often engages during the last four weeks of pregnancy. This is the result of good tonus of the uterine and abdominal muscles. In the multigravida, engagement of the fetal head can happen at any time from week 36, but often only occurs during labour. The nurse or caregiver will determine engagement by means of abdominal palpation.

Descent occurs during the whole course of labour and is especially pronounced during the second stage of labour. Descent indicates that the fetus is progressing through the birth canal. The station of the fetal head is the relationship between the lowest bony part on the presenting part and an imaginary line drawn between the two spinae ischii. When the presenting part of the fetal skull (bony part, not caput succedaneum) or the breech, in cases of a breech presentation, is situated on this imaginary line, the station is 0. This relationship is determined during a vaginal examination.

Level of the head

The concept of determining the level of the fetal head was described by Crichton (1974). It is especially valuable in cases of cephalopelvic disproportion (CPD) with marked moulding of the fetal head. In such cases, determining the station of the fetal head may be misleading (see Figure 6).

This concept is based on dividing the circumference of the round fetal head into fifths. The number of fifths palpable above the symphysis is determined by means of deep pelvic palpation. If the whole fetal head is palpable above the symphysis,

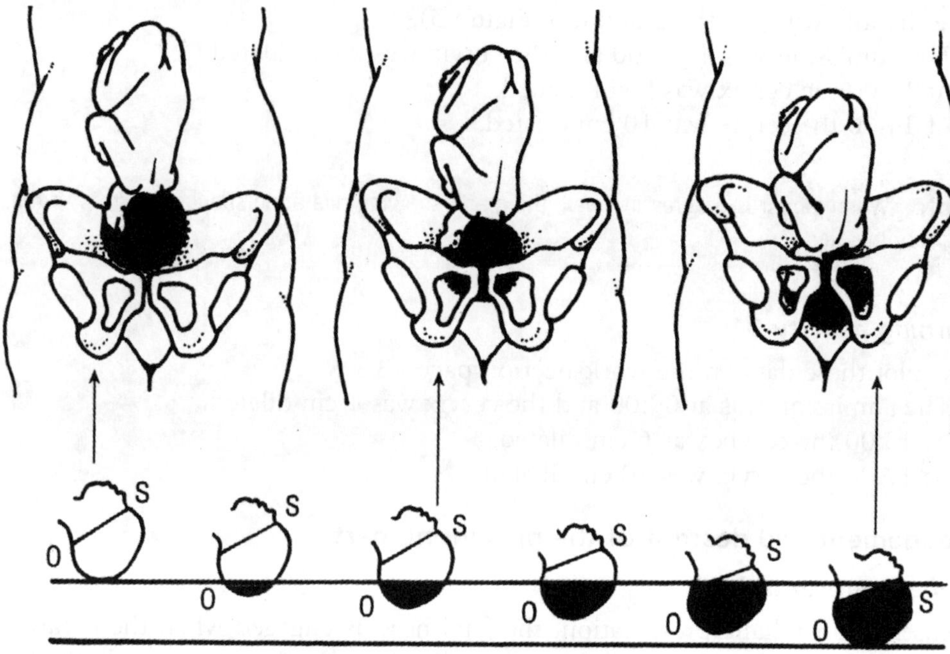

Figure 6 The level of the head (in fifths) above the pubic symphysis

the level of the fetal head is 5/5, if three-fifths of the fetal head are palpable above the symphysis, the level of the fetal head is 3/5.

This concept is especially helpful as:

- in cases of severe moulding of the fetal head, the station of the head may be positive. Because of the severe moulding the largest part of the fetal head is, however, still situated above the pelvic inlet. If the level of the head had been determined, it would have been obvious that 3/5 or more of the fetal head was still palpable above the symphysis.
- the progress of labour can be determined to a certain extent. It is obvious that there is a relationship between station, engagement, descent and level of the presenting part. In normal circumstances engagement denotes a station of –1 with a level of 3/5. A station of 0 implies a level of 2/5. However, if moulding occurs, or a malposition is present, this relationship is no longer valid. In these cases the level of the head is the safer method to use.

Example: Plotting engagement of the fetal head

On the left side of the graph in Figure 7 you will see the words 'Descent of head', with numbers from 0 to 5. Engagement of the fetal head is plotted by means of a circle (O) on the graph.

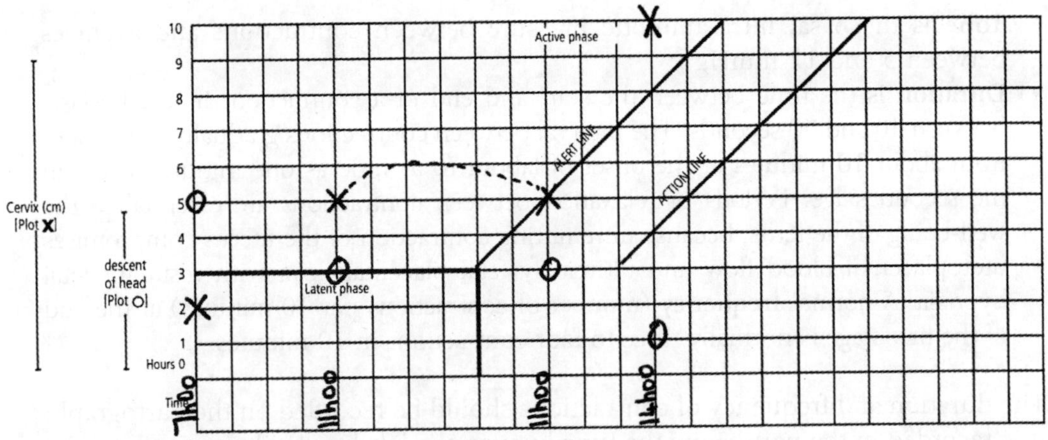

Figure 7 Plotting engagement of the fetal head

Note the following on the graph above:

- The admission was at 07:00. The cervix was 2 cm dilated and the head was 5/5 above the brim.
- At 11:00 the cervix was 5 cm dilated and the head was 3/5 above the brim.
- At 14:00 the cervix was 10 cm dilated and the head 1/5 above the brim.

Important aspects to consider

- Measuring the engagement of the fetal head helps the midwife to follow the progress of labour.
- An abdominal examination must always be done before a vaginal examination.
- The level of the presenting part is therefore determined every time a vaginal examination is being done.

Learning activity 4

Plot these data on the worksheet on page 48.

- The admission was at 16:00. The cervix was 1 cm dilated and the head was 4/5 above the brim.
- At 20:00 the cervix was 4 cm dilated and the head was 3/5 above the brim.
- At 00:00 the cervix was 9 cm dilated and the head 1/5 above the brim.

OBSERVATION OF UTERINE CONTRACTIONS

The following characteristics of contractions should be observed:

- The **intensity** of the uterine contractions is greater in the fundus towards the lower segment. In established labour the intensity of the contraction causes a rise in intra-amniotic pressure to between 25 and 60 mmHg above the basal tone.

- **Tone** is the basal intra-amniotic pressure between contractions and averages between 5 and 12 mmHg.
- **Duration** is the time between the start and end of a contraction. It usually lasts between 40 and 50 seconds. The interval between contractions gradually diminishes from about 10 minutes at the onset of labour to as little as one minute or less in the second stage. Periods of relaxation between contractions are essential to the well-being of the fetus, because unremitting contraction of the uterus compromises uteroplacental blood flow and ultimately fetal placental flow, with resultant fetal hypoxia. A normal **frequency** (number of contractions per 10 minutes) at the end of the first stage is normally three to four contractions in 10 minutes.

The duration and frequency of contractions should be recorded on the partograph. It is recorded in the part below the time line; on the left-hand side you will see the words 'Contractions in 10 mins' (see Figure 9).

The number of contractions per 10 minutes (frequency) is recorded by shading the appropriate number of blocks, for example, if there are two contractions in 10 minutes, two blocks are shaded. The duration of the contractions is marked by shading the blocks in different ways. The key below shows the three ways in which the duration of contractions is recorded on a partograph.

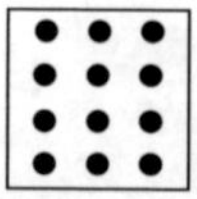

Dots represent mild contractions of less than 20 seconds in duration.

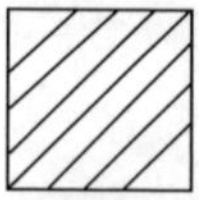

Diagonal lines indicate moderate contractions of 20 to 40 seconds in duration.

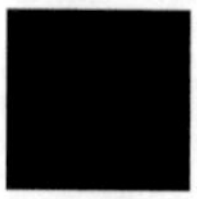

Solid colour indicates strong contractions of longer than 40 seconds in duration.

According to the *Guidelines for Maternity Care in South Africa* (2002) contractions should be assessed two-hourly during the latent stage and half-hourly during the active stage.

Example: Plotting uterine contractions

Figure 9 shows how uterine contractions are plotted on the partograph.

Note the following on the graph:

- Admission was at 11:00. The cervix was 3 cm dilated and the head was 4/5 above the brim. Contractions were two in 10 minutes, each lasting 30 seconds.
- At 15:00 the cervix was 7 cm dilated and the head was 2/5 above the brim. Contractions were four in 10 minutes, each lasting 45 seconds.

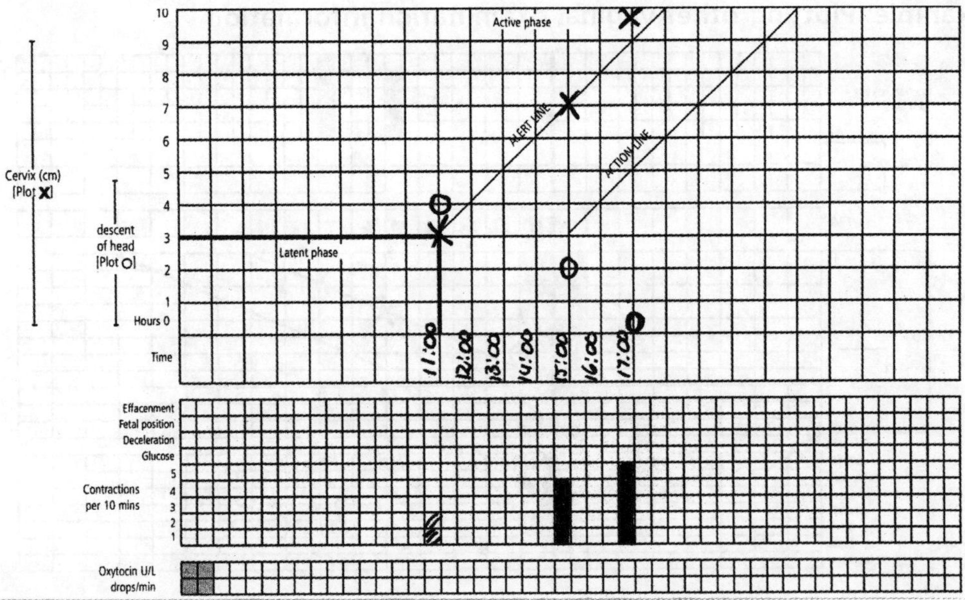

Figure 8 Plotting uterine contractions

- At 17:00 the cervix was 10 cm dilated and the head 0/5 above the brim. Contractions were five in 10 minutes, each lasting 50 seconds.

Learning activity 5

Plot these data on the worksheet on page 49.

- Admission was at 10:00. The cervix was 3 cm dilated and the head was 3/5 above the brim. The contractions were three in 10 minutes, each lasting 30 seconds.
- At 14:00 the cervix was 7 cm dilated and the head was 2/5 above the brim. Contractions were four in 10 minutes, each lasting 40 seconds.
- At 17:00 the cervix was 10 cm dilated and the head 0/5 above the brim. Contractions were five in 10 minutes, each lasting 50 seconds.

Other information from vaginal examinations

Many partographs in South Africa are adapted to include other vaginal examination information that is also valuable for determining the progress of labour. Extra rows of blocks are usually included just below the cervical dilatation section.

The length of the cervix, application, presenting part, position of presenting part and station (descent) of the presenting part are recorded too (see Figure 9).

Example: Plotting other vaginal examination information

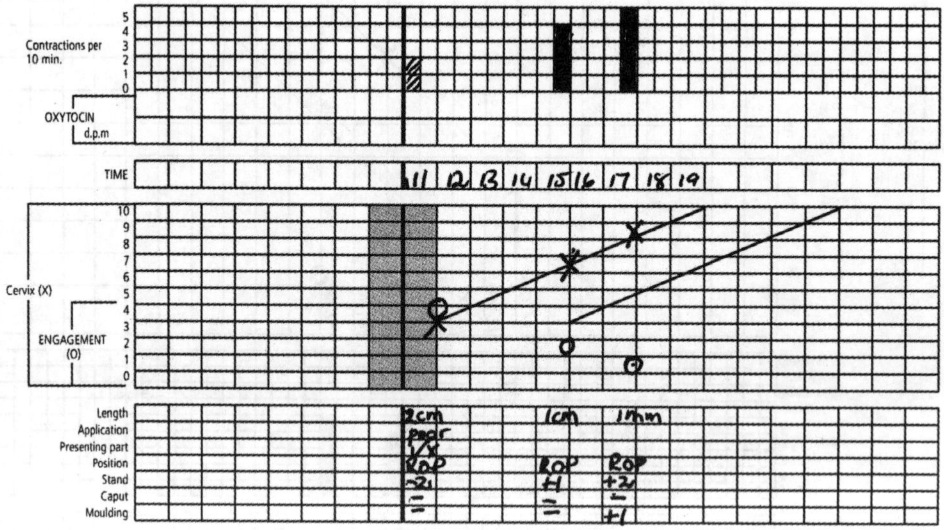

Figure 9 Plotting other vaginal examination information

Note the following on the graph above:

- The admission was at 11:00. The cervix was 3 cm dilated and the head was 4/5 above the brim. The contractions were two in 10 minutes, each lasting 30 seconds. The effacement of the cervix was 2 cm, application is poor, the vertex presents, the fetal head is in a right occipito-posterior position (ROP), no moulding or caput is present, and the station of the head is –2.
- At 15:00 the cervix was 7 cm dilated and the head was 2/5 above the brim. The contractions were 4 in 10 minutes, lasting 40 seconds. The effacement of the cervix is 1 cm, position of the fetal head is ROP, no moulding or caput is present and the station of the head is +1.
- At 17:00 the cervix was 8 cm dilated and the head 1/5 above the brim. The contractions were 5 in 10 minutes, lasting 50 seconds. The effacement of the cervix is 1 mm, the position of fetal head is ROP, moulding is +1 and no caput is present. The station of the head is +2.

Learning activity 6

Plot these data on the worksheet on page 49.

- The admission was at 08:00. The cervix was 3 cm dilated and the head was 4/5 above the brim. The contractions were two in 10 minutes, each lasting 40 seconds. The effacement of the cervix was 2 cm, application is poor, the vertex presents, the fetal head is in a right occipito-anterior position (ROA), no moulding or caput is present and the station of the head is –3.
- At 12:00 the cervix was 8 cm dilated and the head was 2/5 above the brim. The

contractions were three in 10 minutes, lasting 50 seconds. The effacement of the cervix is 0,5 cm, the position of the fetal head is ROA, no moulding or caput is present and the station of the head is 0.

- At 17:00 the cervix was 9 cm dilated and the head 1/5 above the brim. The contractions were four in 10 minutes, lasting 60 seconds. The effacement of the cervix is 1 mm, the position of the fetal head is ROA, moulding is +1 and no caput is present. The station of the head is +1.

OBSERVATION OF THE FETAL CONDITION

Fetal condition during labour can be assessed by obtaining information about the fetal heart rate and patterns, as well as the liquor (amniotic fluid).

The fetal heart rate

The fetal heart rate may be assessed intermittently by means of a monaural (Pinard) stethoscope or handheld Doppler device, or it may be assessed continuously using Electronic Fetal Monitoring (EFM).

The fetal heart rate should be taken over a complete minute in order to listen for beat-to-beat variation. The baseline rate should be between 110 and 160 beats per minute (b.p.m.). Doppler apparatus can be used throughout a contraction, but listening with a Pinard stethoscope during a contraction is uncomfortable for the woman. In addition, fetal heart sounds may be inaudible. The midwife can use a Pinard stethoscope to listen to the fetal heart rate as the contraction is finishing to detect any slow recovery of the fetal heart rate back to the baseline. Normally the baseline rate is maintained during a contraction and immediately after it. However, in late labour some decelerations during contractions with quick recovery are normal and may be due to cord compression or compression of the fetal head. Variability of more than 5 b.p.m. should be maintained throughout labour. If decelerations are heard with a Pinard or Doppler instrument in the first stage of labour, then electronic monitoring may be indicated to assess the extent of decelerations.

Continuous EFM entails the use of electronic apparatus in the form of a fetal heart rate monitor. Continuous recording usually combines a fetal cardiograph and a maternal tocograph in a cardiotocograph (CTG) machine. The CTG provides a graphic record of the response of the fetal heart to uterine activity as well as information about heart rate and variability.

Liquor (amniotic fluid)

Amniotic fluid escapes from the uterus continuously following rupture of the membranes. This fluid should normally remain clear. If the fetus becomes hypoxic, meconium may be passed as hypoxia causes relaxation of the anal sphincter. The amniotic fluid then becomes green as a result of meconium staining. Amniotic fluid that has a muddy yellow colour or is only slightly green may signify a previous event from which the fetus has recovered. It is common and of no significance in post-date babies.

If the fetus is in a breech position, where it is compacted in the pelvis, it may pass meconium because of compression of the abdomen. A fetus in breech position is also prone to fetal compromise and may pass meconium as a result of hypoxia.

The significance of meconium in the amniotic fluid

Until recently the presence of meconium in the amniotic fluid was regarded as a sign of fetal distress. However, the use of a fetal heart monitor during labour and pH sampling of scalp blood has shown that meconium in the amniotic fluid does not necessarily indicate fetal distress. It is nevertheless certain that when there is meconium in the amniotic fluid there is a greater chance that the fetus will be born with a low Apgar score and develop the dangerous meconium-aspiration syndrome. Meconium-stained amniotic fluid is associated with increased neonatal morbidity and even mortality.

There is uncertainty regarding the connection between the colour of meconium and the neonatal prognosis, but it would appear that the presence of thick green meconium before the onset of labour is associated with increased complications.

When meconium is found in the amniotic fluid during labour, it is essential to monitor the fetal heart rate for signs of fetal distress.

Record of the fetal condition

Fetal heart rate, membranes, liquor (amniotic fluid) and moulding of the fetal skull bones give information about how the baby is doing during labour.

- The fetal heart should be auscultated hourly during the latent stage, half-hourly during the active stage and every 15 minutes if fetal distress is suspected.
- Auscultation must be performed before, during and 30 seconds after a contraction.
- Auscultation can also be done using an external mode of the cardiotocograph, if available.
- The fetal heart beat should be assessed **before** artificial rupture of membranes, administration of analgesia or anaesthesia and the administration of other medication. It should be assessed **after** recognition of abnormal uterine activity, alteration in infusion rate of oxytocin, rupture of membranes and other procedures, for example, epidurals, as well as after peak effect time of medication and specifically analgesia.

The **fetal heart rate** is recorded at the top of the partograph. It is recorded every 30 minutes during the active stage. Each square represents 30 minutes. The lines for 120 and 160 b.p.m. are darker to remind the midwife that these are the normal limits of the fetal heart rate.

It is very important to note that the WHO partograph (Figure 10.2) does not make provision for recording decelerations and this should therefore be added. Figure 10.1 is an example of a partograph in which deceleration can be recorded.

Note: Two features of the fetal heart beat should always be assessed, namely:

- the baseline fetal heart rate, that is, the fetal heart rate between contractions, and
- the presence of decelerations and the relation thereof to the contractions.

The **state of the liquor** (amniotic fluid) can assist in assessing fetal condition. Observations of the liquor are to be recorded on the partograph immediately below the fetal heart rate, where indicated on the left-hand side of the partograph. Observations are made with every vaginal examination. They are recorded as:

- I – if the membranes are intact,
- C – if the membranes are ruptured and the liquor is clear, or
- M – if the membranes are ruptured and the liquor is meconium-stained.

Moulding is an important indicator of how well the maternal pelvis will accommodate the fetal head. The following key is used to record moulding:

- 0 – the sutures can be felt easily and the bones are separated,
- + – the bones are just touching each other,
- ++ – the bones are overlapping but can be separated easily with your finger, or
- +++ – the bones are overlapping and cannot be separated with your finger.

Example: Plotting the fetal condition

Note the following on the graphs (see Figures 10A and 10B):

- The fetal heart rate is 130 to 150 b.p.m (Figure 10A + 10B).
- There are no decelerations (Figure 10A + 10B).
- The membranes have ruptured and the liquor is clear (Figure 10A and 10B).
- There is no moulding (Figure 10B).

Note: It is **very important** to remember that increasing moulding with a high head is a sign of cephalopelvic disproportion. **In such cases the patient should be referred to a hospital immediately!**

Learning activity 7

Plot the following data on the worksheet on page 50. Use the same information as for Learning activity 6.

- The fetal heart rate is 150 b.p.m. at 08:00, 130 b.p.m. at 14:00 and 140 b.p.m. at 17:00.
- There are no decelerations.
- The membranes ruptured at 14:00 and the liquor is clear.
- There is +1 moulding and no caput.

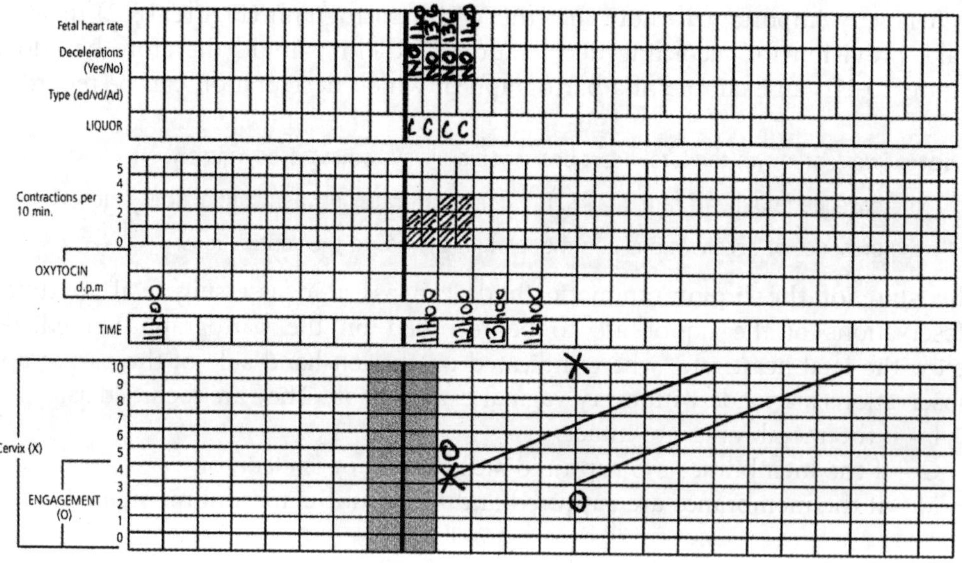

Figure 10A Plotting the fetal condition (including decelerations)

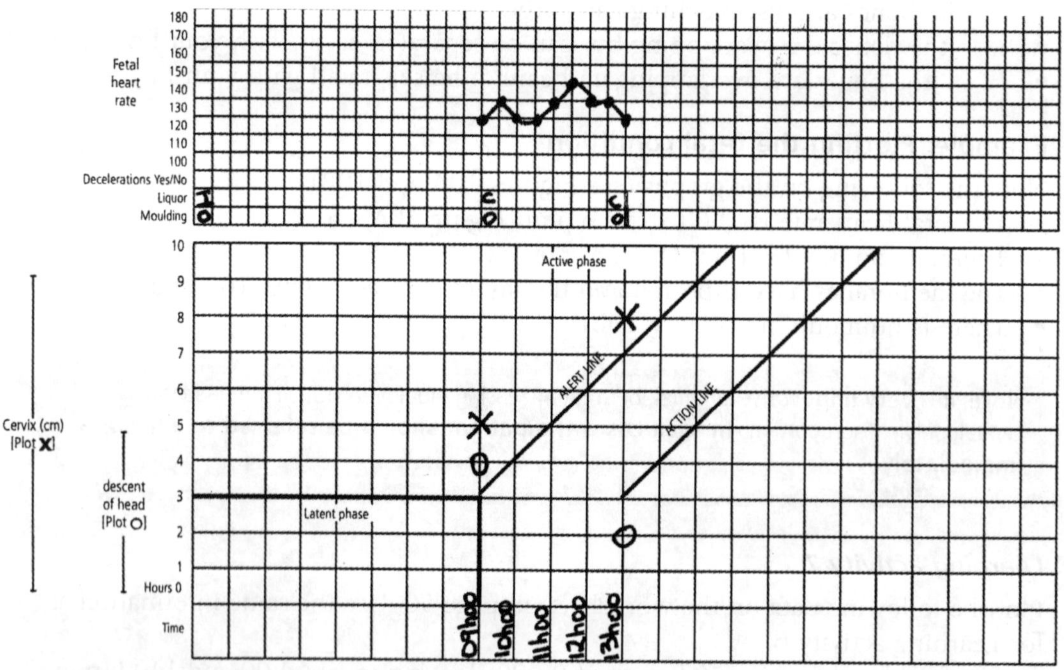

Figure 10B Plotting the fetal condition

OBSERVATION OF THE MATERNAL CONDITION

There are various indicators of maternal condition. All the observations for the mother's condition are written at the bottom of the partograph.

Pulse rate

The pulse rate is a good indicator of the general physical condition of the woman. If the rate increases to more than 100 b.p.m. this may be indicative of anxiety, pain, infection, ketosis or haemorrhage. It is normal practice to record the pulse rate every one to two hours during early labour and every 30 minutes when labour is more advanced.

Temperature

The patient's temperature should remain within the normal range. Pyrexia is indicative of infection or ketosis, or may be associated with epidural analgesia. In normal labour the maternal temperature should be recorded at least every four hours.

Blood pressure

Blood pressure is measured every two to four hour hours unless it is abnormal, in which case more frequent recordings will be necessary, depending on the individual situation. Blood pressure needs to be monitored very closely following epidural or spinal anaesthetic. Hypotension may be caused by the supine position, by shock or as a result of epidural anaesthesia.

Urine analysis

Urine passed during labour should be tested for glucose, ketones and protein. Ketones may occur as a result of starvation or maternal distress when all available energy has been utilised. A low level of ketones is very common during labour and thought not to be significant. Unless a non-diabetic mother has recently eaten a large quantity of carbohydrates or sugar, glucose is normally found in the urine following intravenous administration of glucose.

A trace of protein may be a contaminant following rupture of the membranes, or it may be a sign of increased vaginal mucous discharge or of a urinary infection, but more significant proteinuria may indicate pre-eclampsia.

Fluid balance

A record should be kept of all urine passed to ensure that the bladder is being emptied. If an intravenous infusion is in progress, the fluids administered must be recorded accurately.

The following observations are recorded (see Figure 11):

- **Pulse, blood pressure and temperature** should be recorded every two to four hours, and more frequently if necessary. The *Guidelines for Maternity Care*

in South Africa (2002) prescribe that maternal blood pressure should be taken hourly during the active stage and the pulse rate should be taken half-hourly.
- A rise in temperature accompanied by an increase in pulse rate may indicate maternal dehydration and exhaustion.
- Should the diastolic pressure rise by 10 mmHg and/or the systolic pressure by 15 mmHg, a doctor must be informed.
- An increased pulse rate and a drop in blood pressure may indicate bleeding.

- **Urine output** must be monitored and each sample of urine must be tested for **glucose**, **ketones**, **protein** and **blood**. The mother should be asked to empty her bladder two- to four-hourly.
- **Drugs and rehydration fluids** should be recorded when they were given.
- There is a separate column for recording **oxytocin** given. This appears above the column for rehydration fluids and drugs.

All entries are recorded in the appropriate place on the time line at the time at which the observations are made.

Note the following entries at 10:00 on the graph:
- The observations of the mother are: pulse 70 b.p.m., temperature 37 °C, blood pressure (BP) 110/80 mmHg.

Example: Plotting the maternal condition

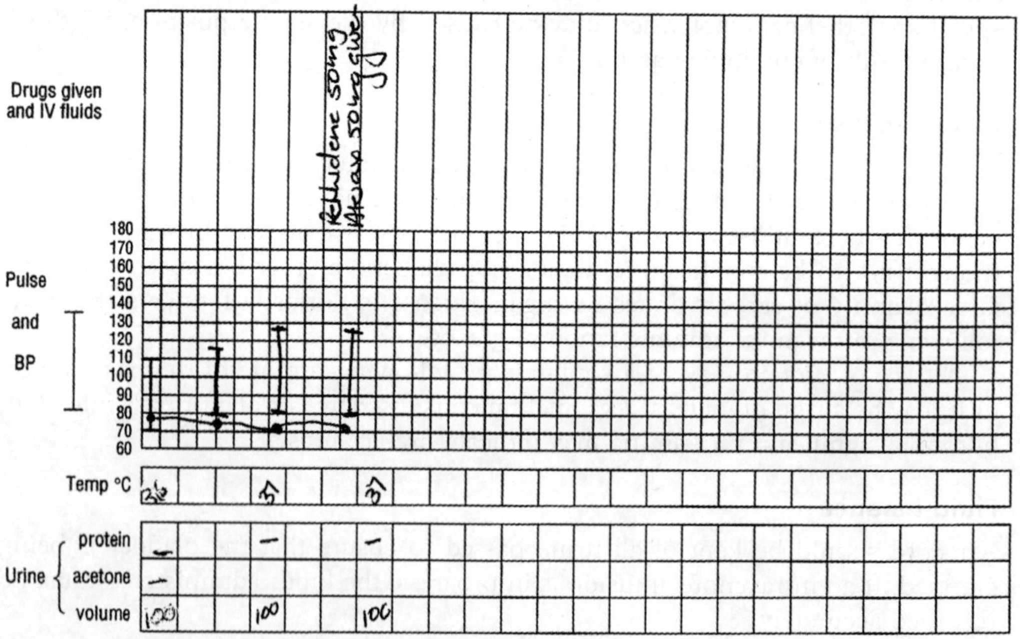

Figure 11 Plotting the maternal condition

- She has passed 100 ml urine containing no abnormal substances.
- She has received 50 mg Pethidine and 50 mg Aterax.
- An IV infusion with 5 U of oxytocin is running at a speed of 15 drops per minute (d.p.m.).

Learning activity 8

Plot the following data on the worksheet on page 50.

- The observations of the mother are: pulse 90 b.p.m., temperature 36,5 °C, BP 140/90 mmHg.
- She passed 200 ml urine containing no abnormal substances.
- She has received 50 mg Pethidine and 50 mg Aterax.
- An IV infusion with 5 U of oxytocin is running at a speed of 15 d.p.m.

A COMPLETED PARTOGRAPH

Learning activity 9

Figure 12 on page 26 shows a completed partograph. Now plot the following data on the worksheet on page 51. Interpret the completed partograph and write down your findings.

- Admission was at 11:00. The cervix was 2 cm dilated and the head was 4/5 above the brim. Contractions were two in 10 minutes, each lasting 30 seconds. The effacement of the cervix is 2 cm, position of fetal head is ROP, no moulding or caput is present. The fetal heart rate was 140 b.p.m. with no decelerations. The membranes were intact. Maternal blood pressure is 120/80 mmHg, pulse is 80 b.p.m. and temperature 36,5 °C. The mother passed 200 ml urine with no protein, ketones or glucose.
- Maternal and fetal observations between 11:30 and 14:30 were as follows:

	Fetus		**Mother**
Time	**Heart rate**	**Decelerations**	**Contractions**
11:30	136	No	2 in 10 minutes, each lasting 30 seconds
12:00	136	No	2 in 10 minutes, each lasting 30 seconds
12:30	144	No	2 in 10 minutes, each lasting 20 seconds
13:00	156	No	2 in 10 minutes, each lasting 20 seconds
13:30	140	No	3 in 10 minutes, each lasting 30 seconds
14:00	130	No	3 in 10 minutes, each lasting 30 seconds
14:30	144	No	3 in 10 minutes, each lasting 30 seconds

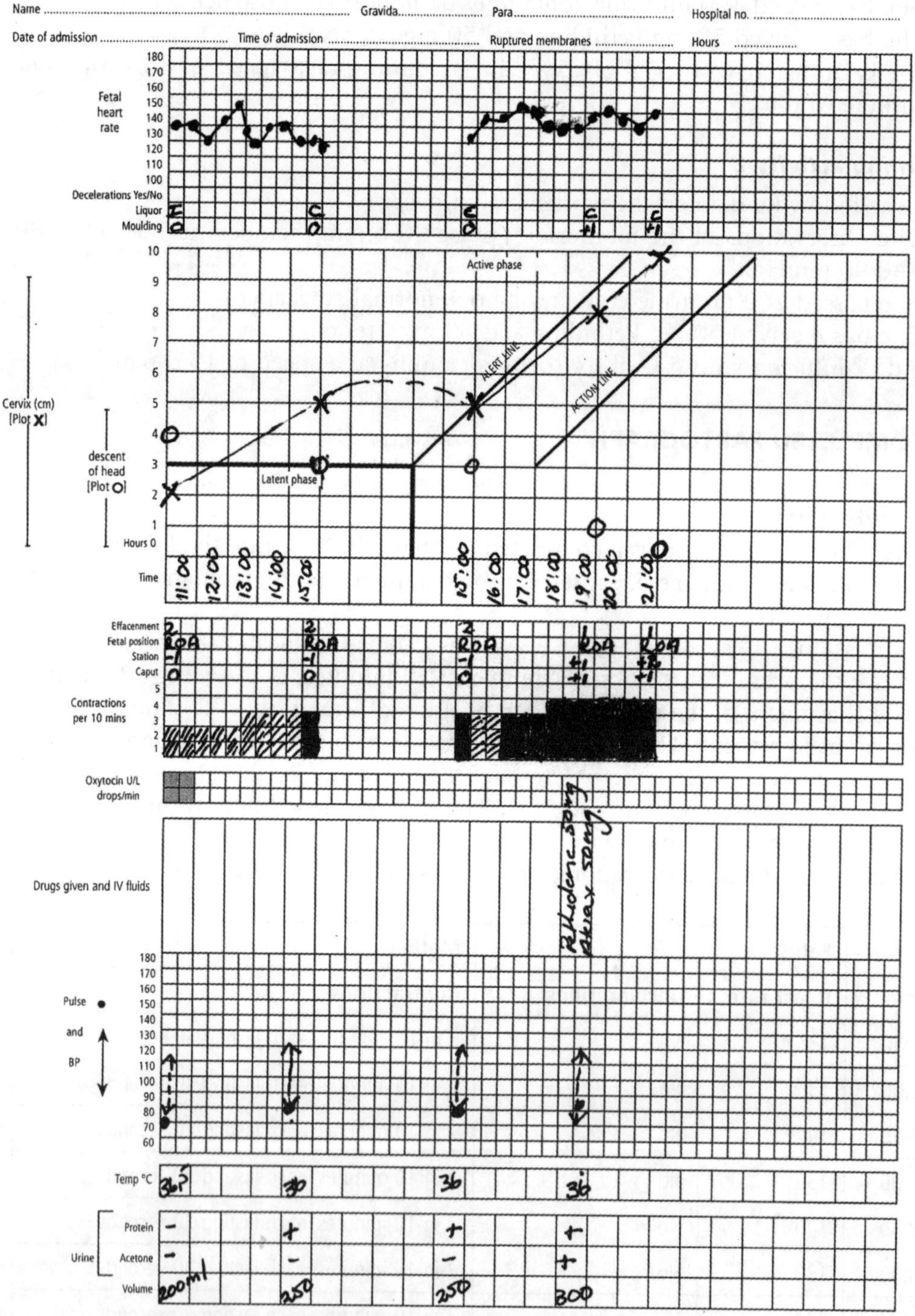

Figure 12 A completed partograph

- At 15:00 the cervix was 5 cm dilated and the head was 3/5 above the brim. The contractions were three in 10 minutes, each lasting 40 seconds. The effacement of the cervix is 1 cm, the position of fetal head is ROP, no moulding or caput is present. The fetal heart rate was 150 b.p.m. with no decelerations. The membranes ruptured spontaneously and the liquor was clear. Maternal blood pressure was 130/70 mmHg, pulse was 74 b.p.m. and temperature was 36 °C. The mother passed 250 ml urine with +protein, no ketones and no glucose.

	Fetus		**Mother**
Time	**Heart rate**	**Decelerations**	**Contractions**
15:30	136	No	3 in 10 minutes, each lasting 30 seconds
16:00	136	No	3 in 10 minutes, each lasting 40 seconds
16:30	144	No	3 in 10 minutes, each lasting 40 seconds
17:00	156	No	3 in 10 minutes, each lasting 30 seconds
17:30	140	No	3 in 10 minutes, each lasting 30 seconds
18:00	130	No	4 in 10 minutes, each lasting 40 seconds
18:30	144	No	4 in 10 minutes, each lasting 40 seconds

- At 19:00 the cervix was 8 cm dilated and the head 1/5 above the brim. The contractions were five in 10 minutes, lasting 50 seconds. The effacement of the cervix is 1 mm, the position of fetal head is ROP, there is + moulding and no caput is present. The fetal heart rate was 150 b.p.m. with no decelerations. The liquor was clear. Maternal blood pressure was 130/80 mmHg, pulse rate 80 b.p.m. and temperature 36 °C. The mother passed 300 ml urine with + protein, + ketones and no glucose. Pethidine 50 mg and Aterax 50 mg were administered to the mother for pain.

	Fetus		**Mother**
Time	**Heart rate**	**Decelerations**	**Contractions**
19:30	136	No	5 in 10 minutes, each lasting 50 seconds
20:00	136	No	5 in 10 minutes, each lasting 60 seconds
20:30	144	No	5 in 10 minutes, each lasting 60 seconds

- At 20h45 the cervix was 10 cm dilated and the head 0/5 above the brim. Contractions were 5 in 10 minutes, each lasting 60 seconds. The effacement of the cervix is 1 mm, the position of fetal head is ROP, moulding is + and no caput is present. The fetal heart rate was 150 b.p.m. with no decelerations. The liquor was clear.

CHAPTER TWO

Prevention and management of prolonged and obstructed labour using the partograph

DEFINITION OF PROLONGED LABOUR

Prolonged labour usually means that progress is *slower* than normal (delayed), or that there is *no* progress (arrest). Thus prolonged labour means an abnormally prolonged *active stage* of labour, when rapid dilatation of the cervix should be taking place. The diagnosis is not associated with a time factor, but rather with the progress of labour as indicated by the tempo of dilatation of the cervix.

It is accepted that a multipara ought to dilate at 1,5 cm per hour and a primigravida at 1 cm per hour. In the normal active stage of labour a dilatation tempo of 1 cm per hour is considered normal. This tempo of dilatation is indicated as such in the cervicogram area of the partograph.

THE RULE OF Ps

There are several causes of prolonged labour and often more than one cause is responsible. For practical purposes the causes can be divided into four groups.

- abnormality of uterine contractions (**Powers**)
- abnormality of the fetus (**Passenger**)
- abnormality of the birth canal, which includes the bony pelvis and the soft tissue structures (**Passage**)
- abnormalities relating to the woman (**Patient**).

These groupings of causes are known as the rule of Ps (or the four Ps) and when a caregiver is confronted by prolonged labour, the cause is sought in one or more of these groups of causes.

Although the groupings are useful, the caregiver should realise that certain causes affect only one or two stages of labour, while others will affect all three stages. For example, cervical stenosis will affect only the first stage of labour, while hypotonic uterine muscle function may affect all three stages.

Abnormality of uterine contractions (Powers)

Abnormal uterine function may cause a **prolonged latent stage**. However, a prolonged latent stage may be followed by a normal active stage.

Abnormal uterine function may also cause a **prolonged active stage** and a prolonged second stage of labour. The contractions may be either inadequate or ineffective. Inadequate contractions last less than 40 seconds and/or are fewer than two in 10 minutes. Ineffective contractions may be adequate, but there is no progress of labour, with no signs of disproportion.

Abnormalities of the fetus (Passenger)

- Abnormalities of position, for example, **occipito-posterior position**, can cause a prolonged first and second stage of labour.
- Abnormalities of presentation, for example, **brow presentation**, **compound presentation**, **face presentation** and **breech presentation** may cause prolonged first and second stages.
- Abnormalities of lie, for example, **oblique** or **transverse** lies, are associated with prolonged labour if the condition is not diagnosed.
- Abnormalities of fetal body size can also cause prolonged labour. A very **large fetus** (more than 4 000 g) may cause a prolonged first stage because of cephalopelvic disproportion. The head is big and moulding is often difficult. A prolonged first stage is common in this case.
- Associated factors in the mother that adversely affect the labour process include being overweight, as well as diabetes mellitus and hypotension. Prolonged labour in this type of woman worsens the outcomes for mother and fetus.
- Congenital abnormalities of the fetus, for example, **hydrocephalus**, **congenital ascites**, **congenital polycystic kidneys**, **tumours of the liver** and **siamese twins** may also lead to prolonged first and second stages of labour.

Abnormalities of the birth canal (Passage)

- Abnormalities of the bony pelvis, for example, of the **pelvic inlet**, **mid-pelvis** and **pelvic outlet** may cause prolonged labour.
- Abnormalities of the soft tissue of the birth canal may sometimes cause prolonged labour.
- **Atresia** of the vulva caused by congenital or acquired conditions may cause prolonged labour, especially during the second stage.
- **Vaginal atresia**, **septa** or **cysts** may cause prolonged labour even after vaginoplasty.
- During assessment of the **cervix**, it must be determined whether or not the patient is really in labour. The *diagnosis of labour* is based on painful contractions plus one of three factors: a sign ('show') of labour, spontaneous rupture of membranes and/or complete intake of the cervix that starts to dilate. After labour induction, the diagnosis is based on one factor only, namely cervical dilatation (3 to 4 cm or more). A patient must really be in labour in order to expect progress.
- **Cervical stenosis** may be of congenital origin or result from cauterisation,

trauma during a delivery, an abortion or after a cone biopsy. The elderly primigravida often has a very rigid cervix.

- **Cervical myomata** of a significant size can also cause prolonged labour.
- **Intramural myomata** of the uterus may cause prolonged labour, because they may also cause abnormal uterine contractions.
- **Other pelvic tumours**, for example, ovarian masses, broad ligament masses or a pelvic kidney may cause prolonged labour by ending up in the pelvic cavity and causing obstruction.
- Other aspects of the birth canal that may cause prolonged labour include the following:
  - The status of the **membranes** across the presenting part is assessed to check whether they are intact or ruptured. With normal progress, intact membranes do not need to be ruptured, whereas they are usually ruptured when poor progress is made.
  - **Application**, that is, how tightly the presenting part is pressing against the cervix, may be assessed. Application is not important between contractions, but during contractions the presenting part should press so tightly against the cervix that it is difficult (sometimes impossible) to insert a finger between it and the cervix. The causes of poor application are false labour, latent stage, inadequate contractions or something that keeps the presenting part high, for example, a large fetus or a small, narrow pelvis.
- Cephalopelvic disproportion can be recognised by the following findings:
  - The head is not engaged in the pelvis (3/5 or more of the head is still palpable above the brim of the pelvis on abdominal examination).
  - There is severe moulding of the fetal skull.

Abnormalities relating to the woman (Patient)

Certain factors in the patient may contribute to prolonged labour:

- A **full bladder** hinders engagement and also tends to lead to a decrease in uterine contractions.
- **Insufficient analgesia** lead to a vicious circle of pain, anxiety and spasms. The catecholamines thus produced tend to cause ineffective uterine contractions. Often when such women receive an epidural anaesthetic, they progress remarkably well.
- **Dehydration** may cause ineffective uterine contractions. A woman normally requires approximately 1 litre of fluids per 6 to 8 hours. Dehydration can be diagnosed by observing the patient's intake and secretion chart. The urine of dehydrated women will be concentrated, the patient's tongue will become dry and acidosis may eventually set in, with ketonuria as well as fever.
- The **supine hypotensive syndrome** may diminish uterine contractions.
- The woman's psyche may play an important role in her progress in labour. A **negative attitude** towards pregnancy, labour or the staff may affect progress adversely.

- **Inadequate pain relief** can lead to poor progress in labour. Excessive pain leads to fear, which may then aggravate the pain. The result is the secretion of catecholamines, which cause irregular and ineffective uterine contractions.
- The maternal position may have an influence.

CARE OF WOMEN IN PROLONGED LABOUR

The principles of care for a woman in prolonged labour are:
- finding the cause (4 Ps or rule of Ps),
- treating the abnormalities, if possible,
- re-evaluating the progress of labour two- to four-hourly, and
- giving normal basic care during labour.

The first step is to establish the cause of prolonged labour using the rule of Ps. A caesarean section is performed immediately if prolonged labour is the result of a condition that could not be prevented or will endanger either the mother or the fetus. An example of such a condition would be cephalopelvic disproportion without progress.

If the condition is one in which progress may be possible, especially with specific management, for example, hypotonic uterine function, labour is allowed to progress with very good control and purposeful management.

General precautions include the following:
- The vital signs of the mother such as pulse, blood pressure, temperature and urine output are carefully monitored, as are signs of exhaustion.
- The mother needs to take in adequate fluids and kilojoules to ensure that she does not become dehydrated or ketonic.
- Adequate pain relief and sedation is absolutely essential when prolonged labour is expected. In these cases epidural anaesthetic is very effective and may even have a direct therapeutic effect (for example, in the case of hypertonic uterine function).
- The woman and her partner have certain expectations regarding the duration of labour. If the normal duration of labour extends beyond this period, tension and anxiety increase. The woman begins to doubt her own ability to cope with the situation. It is important to keep the woman and her husband informed about the progress of labour and the reasons why she is not progressing as anticipated, for example, 'the baby's head must still turn'.
- The fetal status must be monitored carefully. Where facilities exist, electronic and chemical methods will be very valuable. Where these facilities are not available, the fetal heart rate must be monitored every 15 minutes before, during and after a contraction.
- The regular assessment of the progress of labour is clearly the most important aspect in the successful and effective management of prolonged labour.

Although an abdominal examination to establish the level of the vertex above the pubic symphysis can often indicate progress, dilatation of the cervix is the best method. A vaginal examination should be repeated at least four-hourly, but more often if it appears to be necessary.

- Be alert to meconium in the liquor, as its presence involves an increased risk of intra-uterine infection and asphyxia neonatorium.
- The bladder must be kept empty.

BASIC MIDWIFERY CARE DURING PROLONGED LABOUR

Mobility and position of the patient during the first stage of labour

The woman should be encouraged to remain mobile as long as possible during the first stage of labour, as walking will increase her level of comfort and promote less frequent, more efficient contractions. It also encourages engagement and descent of the presenting part, while serving to distract the woman's attention from the discomfort of her contractions.

Women should not be nursed in a dorsal position during labour. When women lie on their backs, this leads to diminished uteroplacental blood flow, resulting in fetal distress, as well as decreased blood flow to the maternal kidneys, with a reduction in urinary excretion, which can cause oedema. Supine hypotension syndrome may also occur.

When backache occurs, as in the case of posterior positions of the occiput, it is usually caused by pressure of the presenting part on the sacrum, which refers pain to the lower back. Positioning can facilitate rotation and promote maternal comfort and relaxation.

Maternal positioning can also be used to prevent or correct malposition of the fetus. An all-fours or side-lying position, combined with the pelvic rocking motion, may be used to turn an occipito posterior fetus to a more favourable position. Another position that may help with rotation of an occipito-posterior position is the lunge. It widens the side of the pelvis towards which the mother is lunging. Positions such as prolonged lying on the back or semi-seated positions, and even prolonged side-lying, may impede rotation and progress in labour. Frequent position changes appear to be effective in facilitating fetal rotation and descent.

The patient should be encouraged to adopt whatever position she finds comfortable during the first stage of labour. Many patients will choose upright positions to begin with and then adopt lateral recumbent positions as labour becomes more advanced.

Position changes are sometimes helpful in alleviating mild fetal distress, if the distress is due to supine hypotension syndrome or cord compression.

Augmentation of labour

The most common methods for augmentation of labour are also methods for induction of labour, namely amniotomy and administering an IV oxytocin infusion. Breast nipple stimulation may also be effective, together with ambulation (walking) and position changes.

When uterine activity is insufficient to produce progressive cervical dilatation, an amniotomy may be performed if the patient is in active labour. Amniotomy is thought to release arachidonic acid, a precursor of prostaglandins, which enhance uterine activity. It also promotes the descent of the presenting part, thus applying pressure on the cervix, which further stimulates contractions. Available data suggest that an amniotomy will shorten the length of spontaneous labour and may forestall the need for oxytocin infusion in some women. The combination of amniotomy with oxytocin may provide a better stimulation of labour than oxytocin alone (Enkin *et al*, 2000:338).

Membranes can be ruptured if the women is in active labour and the fetal head is 3/5 and less above the brim of the pelvis. However, mother-to-child transmission of HIV is more likely with than without ruptured membranes. It should therefore be a contra-indication in HIV-positive women.

Labour may be augmented by an IV infusion of oxytocin. Lower dosages and lower rates will be required than with induction of labour. Oxytocin is a potentially dangerous preparation and individuals can react very differently to the same dosage. It is, therefore, advisable to begin with a very low dosage and to increase it gradually until good contractions are obtained. Various methods of intravenous administration are used, but it is advisable to use two containers. Two units of oxytocin are added to one container, which is connected to the main infusion. The main infusion contains only IV fluid without oxytocin. Caregivers should remember that the dosage rates of the oxytocin infusion and the patient's requirements for fluids and kilojoules are totally different.

Augmentation of labour by oxytocin according to *Guidelines for Maternity Care in South Africa* (2002)

1. Add two units of oxytocin to 1 litre of Ringer's lactate.
2. Start infusion at a rate of 15 d.p.m. (60 ml per hour).
3. Increase by 15 d.p.m. every 30 minutes until a minimum of three strong contractions in 10 minutes are achieved.
4. The infusion rate should not exceed 60 d.p.m.
5. Contractions, pulse rate, fetal heart beat, blood pressure and breathing should be monitored.
6. If the contractions become too strong or too frequent or too long, the rate of the infusion should be decreased.

Note: The rate of oxytocin should **not** be increased if the woman is already experiencing strong contractions. The strength of the contractions should be determined according to the general progress of labour. In other words, it is not normal for a woman to get four strong contractions of 60 seconds each if she is only 4 cm dilated.

If the oxytocin is administered by means of an infusion pump this ensures that it flows at an absolutely uniform speed. If a cardiotocograph is available, it is advisable to use it to monitor labour. The maximum frequency of uterine contractions is five contractions in 10 minutes. The contractions should last no longer than 60 seconds and the resting tone should not rise higher than 22 mmHg (preferably less than 15 mmHg). The oxytocin infusion must be stopped immediately if:

- hypertonic uterine contractions occur, or
- the pattern of the fetal heart beat becomes abnormal.

Contra-indications for the use of oxytocin

The following are contra-indications for the use of oxytocin:

- evidence of disproportion, for example, moulding of +3,
- any patient with a scar in the uterus,
- when the presenting part is not vertex,
- grand multiparity, and
- when there is fetal distress.

Note: It is **very important** that oxytocin should not be administered without a doctor's prescription or very well developed protocols in the unit.

Prevention of ketoacidosis and maternal exhaustion

The patient should receive sufficient fluids and kilojoules to prevent maternal exhaustion, which can result in ketosis or ketoacidosis. The vigorous muscle contractions of the uterus during labour demand a continuous supply of glucose. If this is not obtained from the diet the body will start to metabolise protein and fat stores in an effort to provide glucose (gluconeogenesis), without which uterine muscle inertia will set in. Maternal ketoacidosis will result in fetal acidosis, fetal distress and ineffective uterine contractions, causing prolonged labour, poor co-operation from the mother in the second stage, and the possibility of postpartum bleeding.

This means that women should be allowed to eat and drink as and when they require to during labour. Patients will usually take in some food during the latent stage, but will limit their intake automatically during the active stage.

During labour, women need energy, which can be supplied by the intake of carbohydrates. A woman should take in foods that are easily absorbed, particularly foods that are low in fat and roughage. However, only small amounts should be eaten at a time.

The opinion that food and drink should be withheld once labour has commenced is still widely held. However, there is an equally strong view that, except in the case of patients at high risk of needing general anaesthesia, the benefits of allowing patients nourishment as they wish far outweigh the benefits of more restricted policies.

Policies that restrict oral intake during labour have the objective of reducing the risk of regurgitation and inhalation of acid gastric contents during the use of general anaesthesia. Aspirated contents from the stomach may contain undigested food and predispose the patient to airway obstruction. However, if the woman has not eaten during labour, the strongly acidic gastric juice can cause a chemical pneumonitis if inhaled (Mendelson's syndrome).

There is no guarantee that withholding food and drink during labour will ensure that the stomach will be empty in the event that general anaesthesia should become necessary. Nor can fasting during labour be relied on to lower the acidity of the gastric contents.

Patients can be advised in advance to bring hard sweets they can suck, as well as sweet cooldrinks or fruit juices. This simultaneously provides the necessary energy and fluid. A practice that patients have found acceptable is to wrap a piece of ice in gauze for them to suck. This enables the woman to keep her lips and throat moist without the danger of inadvertent aspiration of ice or large gulps of water.

A common response to the problem of dehydration or ketosis is administering an intravenous infusion of glucose and fluid. The effect of this practice should be carefully weighed against the alternative course of allowing patients to eat and drink as they desire.

Intravenous infusion of carbohydrate-containing solutions can cause an increase in plasma glucose levels in the fetus, but may also result in a decrease in umbilical arterial blood pH. Latrogenic hyperinsulinism can occur in the fetus in reaction to the increased fetal blood glucose levels when patients receive more than 25 g of glucose intravenously during labour. This can result in neonatal hypoglycaemia within two hours of the baby's birth. There is also evidence that these babies develop a greater level of jaundice than those whose mothers were given less glucose.

An IV infusion is always a good choice in the case of prolonged labour. Once prolonged labour has been diagnosed, it is advisable to keep the patient nil per os.

Pain relief

Non-pharmacological methods

Non-pharmacological pain relief methods may be used either instead of or in addition to analgesia. These techniques remove or diminish the painful stimulus at the source, or provide powerful alternate stimuli to compete with and inhibit pain awareness, or reduce the woman's negative mental, emotional and physical reaction to pain. Examples are different ways of distraction, the midwife's relationship with the patient, attendance by significant others and doulas, breathing exercises, relaxation techniques, teaching the patient about pain, maternal position changes, localised pressure to reduce back pain, superficial heat and cold, massage of the lower back and hot baths and showers.

Pharmacological methods

Both analgesics (which cause a decreased awareness of pain without loss of consciousness) and anaesthesia (the partial or complete loss of sensation with or without loss of consciousness) may be used to reduce pain during the intrapartum period. Sedatives (to decrease fear and anxiety) may also be used together with analgesics.

Analgesics

Although the intramuscular injection of analgesics is not ideal, it is a method commonly used during labour. Once the midwife decides to use them, she has to find a compromise between efficient pain relief and possible side effects.

Efficient pain relief often requires such a high dose that side effects are common. These include nausea, vomiting and dizziness in the mother and respiratory suppression in the neonate.

Analgesics should not be given to all women in labour as a matter of course. The midwife should assess each patient as an individual, taking the advantages and disadvantages of such treatment into account. The patient must be consulted and her wishes also considered. Pain relief at the right moment during labour can greatly enhance the emotional satisfaction felt by the mother, while giving it too late in the first stage can result in her being unable to bear down effectively in the second stage, with consequent feelings of guilt. These could, in turn, have an adverse effect on the mother-child relationship, also affecting breast-feeding. Therefore the timing of administration of analgesics is of the utmost importance.

Pethidine and Naloxone

- The most common analgesic preparation is **Pethidine**. The usual dose is 50-100 mg intramuscularly. This is only effective in 50% of patients. Nausea and vomiting also occurs in 50% of patients receiving this medication. Pethidine passes virtually unhindered through the placenta, often affecting the neonate. Suppressed respiration occurs until 48 hours after the delivery in such cases, often accompanied by feeding problems and suppression of certain neuro-behaviourial tests. Caregivers need to bear in mind that the neonate cannot effectively metabolise Pethidine. Its half life in an adult is three hours, while in the neonate it is 22,7 hours.
- **Naloxone** (NarcanR), 200 mg intramuscularly or TV to the mother, will improve breathing, feeding and neuro-behaviourial of the baby response for 48 hours. Its effect in an adult lasts for a limited time, while in the neonate it lasts much longer, again probably as a result of slower metabolism.

Sedatives are often administered with an analgesic, both because the labouring patient is often very tense, and also because they often lessen the incidence of vomiting and nausea caused by Pethidine. The preparation most commonly used with Pethidine is hydroxyzine (Aterax®). Caregivers need to keep in mind that Aterax® potentiates the effect of Pethidine.

RECORDING OBSERVATIONS OF PROLONGED LABOUR ON A PARTOGRAPH

Prolonged latent stage

Learning activity 10

Study Figure 13 on page 38 and answer the questions that follow.

1. Write down your interpretations of this partograph.
2. What are the possible causes for this/these problem(s)?
3. How would you manage this/these problem(s)?

Prolonged active stage

At the action line

If a woman's labour reaches the action line, a decision must be made about the cause of the slow progress and action needs to be taken. The decision as to what action to take to assist labour must be made with a doctor, preferably in a hospital.

Moving to the right of the alert line

In the active stage of labour, plotting of the cervical dilatation will normally remain on, or to the left of the alert line. When dilatation crosses to the right of the alert line, this is a warning sign that labour may be prolonged. When the dilatation moves to the right of the alert line, the mother must be transferred to a hospital, unless she is very near to delivering. The possible reasons for the prolonged labour should be determined.

Learning activity 11

Look at Example A in Figure 1.4 on page 39 and answer the questions that follow. The fetus is in a left occipito-posterior position (LOP).

1. Write down your interpretations of this graph.
2. What are the possible causes for this/these problem(s)?
3. How would you manage this/these problem(s)?

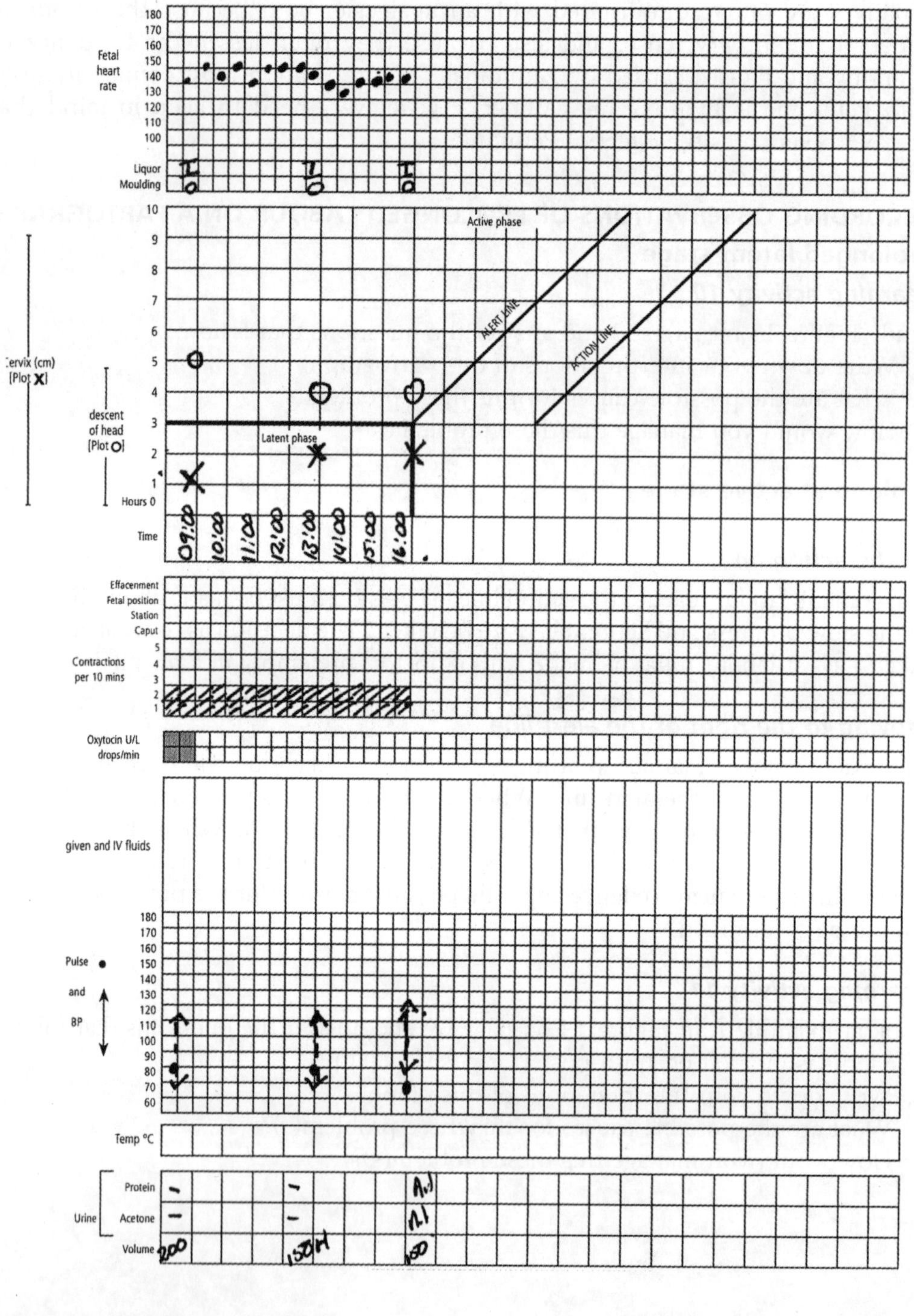

Figure 13 Prolonged latent stage

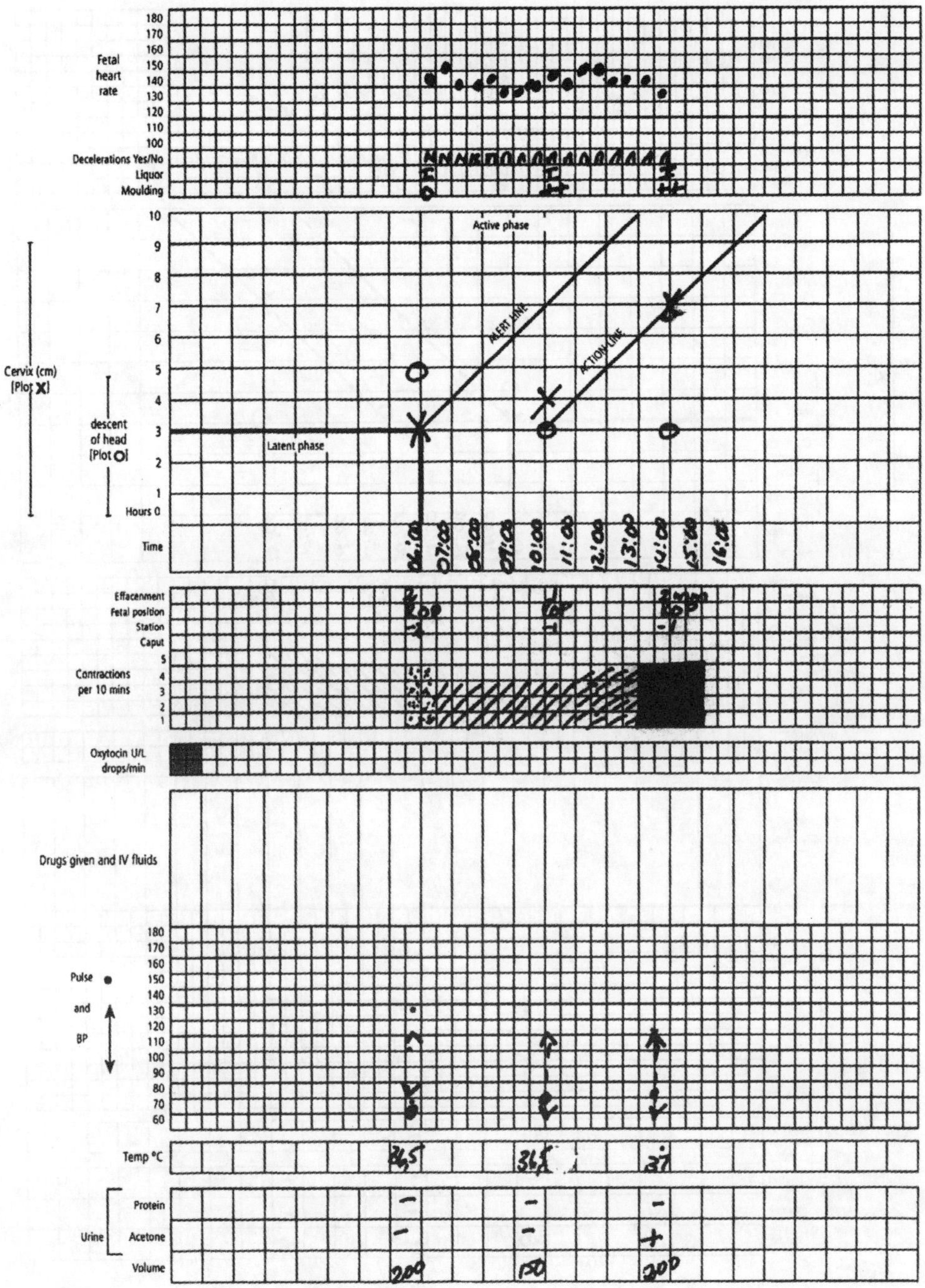

Figure 14 Prolonged active stage (Example A)

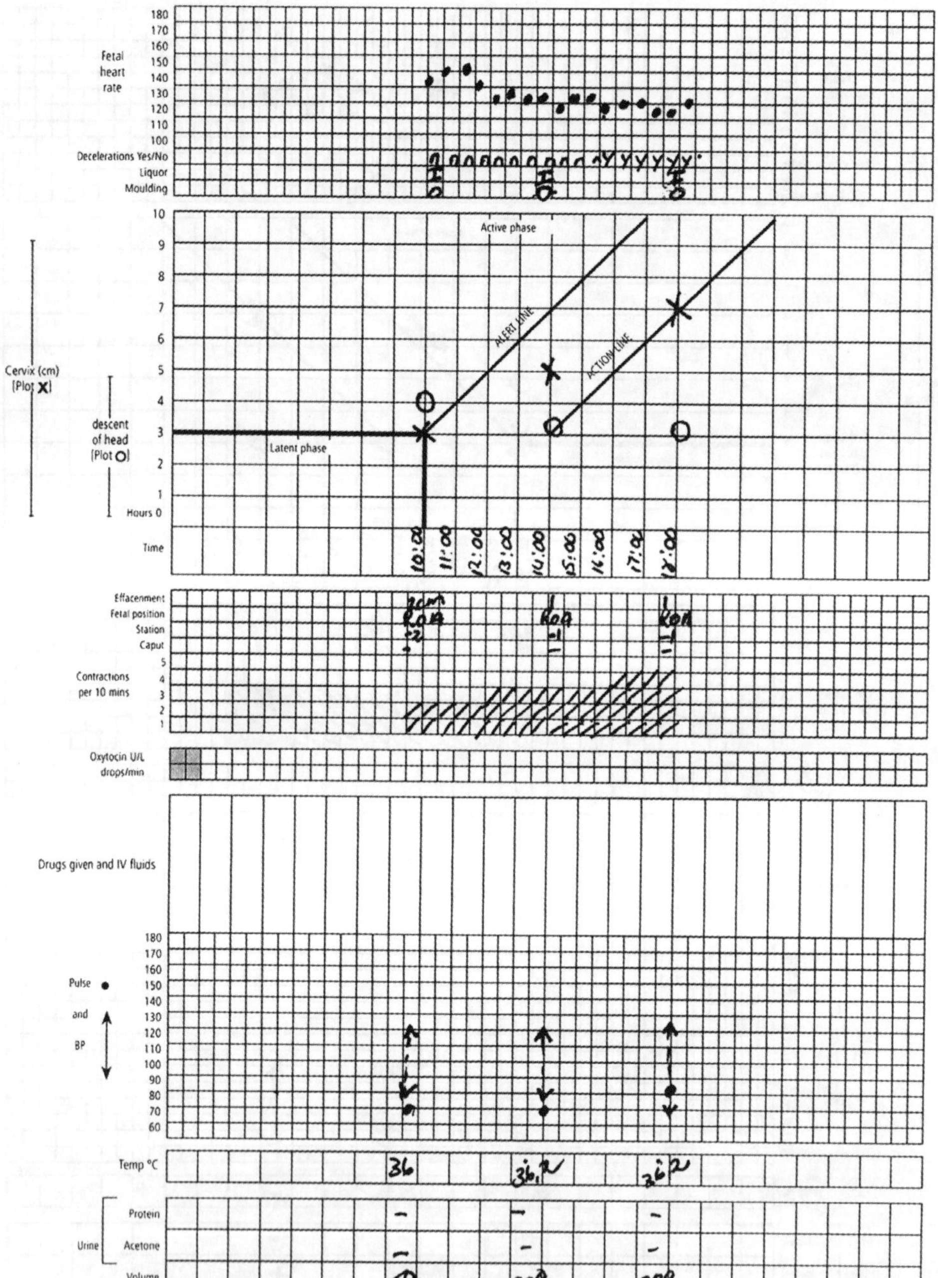

Figure 15 Prolonged active stage (Example B)

Learning activity 12

Look at Example B in Figure 15 on page 40 and answer the questions that follow, particularly at the observations recorded in 10.00. The fetus is in a left occipito-anterior (LOA) position. (Note that LD stands for 'late decelerations'.)

1. What do you think is the most possible reason for prolonged labour in this case?
2. You work in a clinic that is about an hour from the nearest hospital. You have started to arrange for a transfer and are waiting for transport to arrive. Which of the following options would you choose to manage the patient's condition? Motivate why you choose or don't choose each alternative.
   a) Rupture membranes.
   b) Augment labour. How will you do this? Is it in the scope of practice of a midwife to do this?
   c) Ensure adequate maternal hydration and nutrition. What will be most preferable at this point?
   d) Get the patient out of bed and mobilise her in different upright positions.
   e) Give pain relief. What type will be most preferable at this point?

PROLONGED LABOUR: CASE STUDY

Learning activity 13

You work in a midwifery obstetric unit (MOU) that is about one hour from the nearest referral hospital. Benilo, a primigravida, has attended your antenatal clinics regularly from 22 weeks of pregnancy. She experienced no problems during pregnancy. Benilo came to the clinic on 29 March at 03:00 complaining of lower abdominal and back pains. You assess the patient and find the following.

With abdominal palpation:

- She is 40 weeks pregnant.
- The fetus is in an right occipito-anterior position (ROA).
- The head is 3/5 above the brim of the pelvis.
- Fetal heart rate is present at 150 b.p.m.
- The fetus moves well.
- The contractions are three in 10 minutes, last about 30 seconds and are moderately strong.

With a vaginal examination:

- The cervix is 2 cm dilated.
- The cervix is 0,5 cm effaced.
- Application of head is poor.
- Fetal position is ROA.
- Station of the head is 0.

- Membranes are intact.
- No caput or moulding is present.

Maternal vital signs:
- BP is 110/70 mmHg.
- Pulse rate is 90 b.p.m.
- Temperature is 36,9 °C.

Benilo has passed 200 ml urine, which was normal when tested.
She is a little anxious and says she is afraid because she does not know what to expect. The contractions are becoming painful.

1. a) Plot all the above information on the worksheet on page 53.
   b) Write down the conclusions to which you come when you look at the partograph.
   c) Write down the care measures that you would implement for this patient. Motivate your answers.

The protocol in your MOU is to observe the progress of labour two-hourly (abdominal palpation and vaginal examinations). The maternal and fetal observations were taken half-hourly and were normal. When you did the next observation of progress of labour two hours later, at 05:00, they were as follows:

With abdominal palpation:
- The head is 3/5 above the brim of the pelvis.
- The fetal heart rate is 160 b.p.m. with no decelerations.
- The contractions are three in 10 minutes, last about 30 seconds and are moderately strong.

With a vaginal examination:
- The cervix is 3 cm dilated.
- The cervix is 0.5 cm effaced.
- Application of head is poor.
- Fetal position is ROA.
- Station of the head is 0.
- Membranes are intact.
- No caput or moulding is present.

Maternal vital signs:
- BP is 110/70 mmHg.
- Pulse rate is 90 b.p.m.
- Temperature is 36,9 °C.

Benilo says the contractions are now quite sore!

2. a) Plot all the above information on the partograph on page 53.
   b) Write down the conclusions to which you come when you look at the partograph.
   c) Write down the care measures you would implement for this patient. Motivate your answers.

At 07:00, just before day staff came on duty, the observations were as follows:

With abdominal palpation:
- The head is 3/5 above the brim of the pelvis.
- The fetal heart rate is 140 b.p.m. with no decelerations. The fetal heart rate was observed half-hourly and the baseline rate stayed between 140 and 150 b.p.m. with no decelerations.
- The contractions are four in 10 minutes, last about 30 to 40 seconds and are becoming stronger.

With a vaginal examination:
- The cervix is 5 cm dilated.
- The cervix is 0.5 cm effaced.
- Application of head is poor.
- Fetal position is ROA.
- Station of the head is 0.
- Membranes are intact.
- No caput or moulding is present.

Maternal vital signs:
- BP is 120/80 mmHg.
- Pulse rate is 80 b.p.m.
- Temperature is 36,0 °C.

Benilo says the contractions are becoming very painful!

3. a) Plot all the above information on the partograph on page 53.
   b) Write down what you will tell the day staff about the patient when you hand over to them.

When you came on duty that evening at 19:00 you found this information in the partograph (see Figure 16 on pg 44). Study the partograph and answer question 4.

4. a) Write down what observations you make regarding the recordings on the partograph at 09:00 and 11:00.

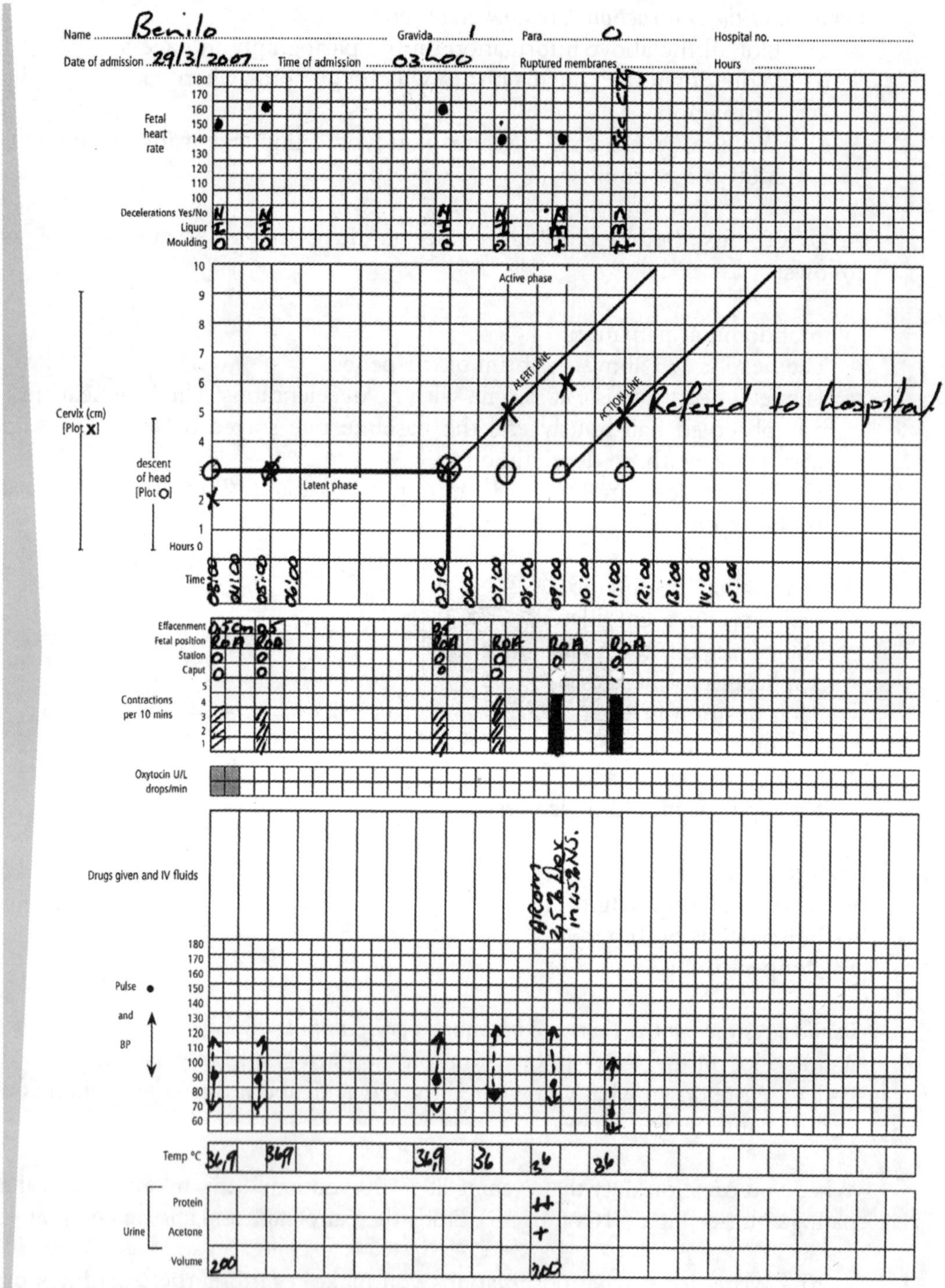

Figure 16 Partograph completed by day staff

b) What are the possible reasons for the prolonged labour?
c) Comment on the way the day staff managed the patient.

SUMMARY

The partograph is a graphic recording of progress of labour to detect labour that is not progressing normally, to indicate when augmentation of labour is appropriate and to recognise cephalopelvic disproportion long before labour becomes obstructed. The partograph assists in early decision on transfer, augmentation and termination of labour. It also increases the quality and regularity of all observations on the fetus and the mother in labour and aids in early recognition of problems with either.

The learner should have obtained the following outcome after completion of this course:

- The learner has developed the knowledge and skills to use the partograph in practice to assess maternal and fetal conditions and the progress of labour and to prevent complications in a timely way, for example, maternal and fetal distress and prolonged or obstructed labour.

Worksheets for learning activities

These partographs are provided for learners to complete the learning activities in this book.

Learning activity 1

Plotting cervical dilatation when the woman is admitted in the latent stage of labour

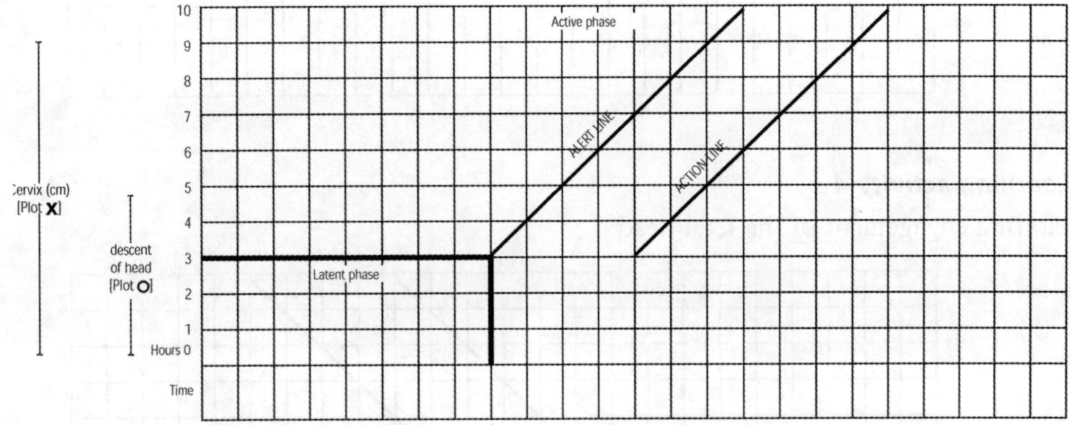

Learning activity 2

Plotting cervical dilatation when the woman is admitted in the active stage of labour

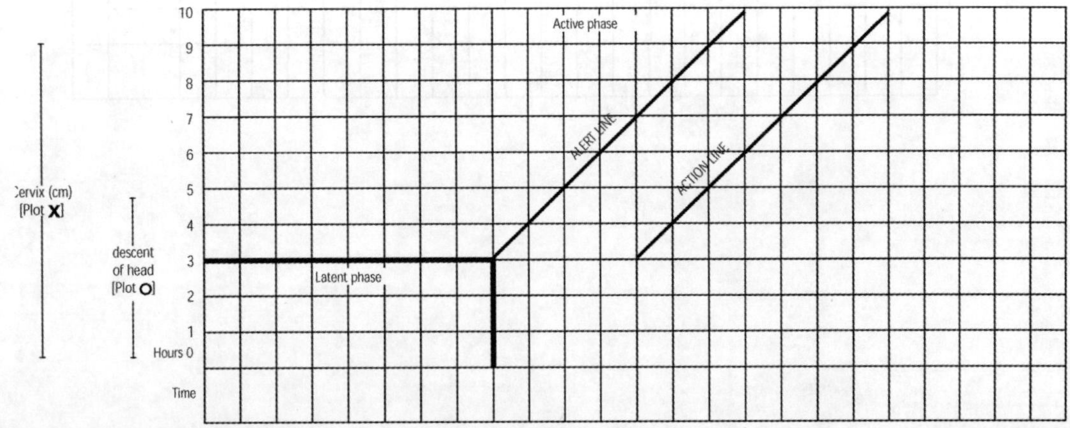

Learning activity 3

Plotting cervical dilatation when the woman is admitted in the latent stage, but proceeds to the active stage before eight hours have elapsed

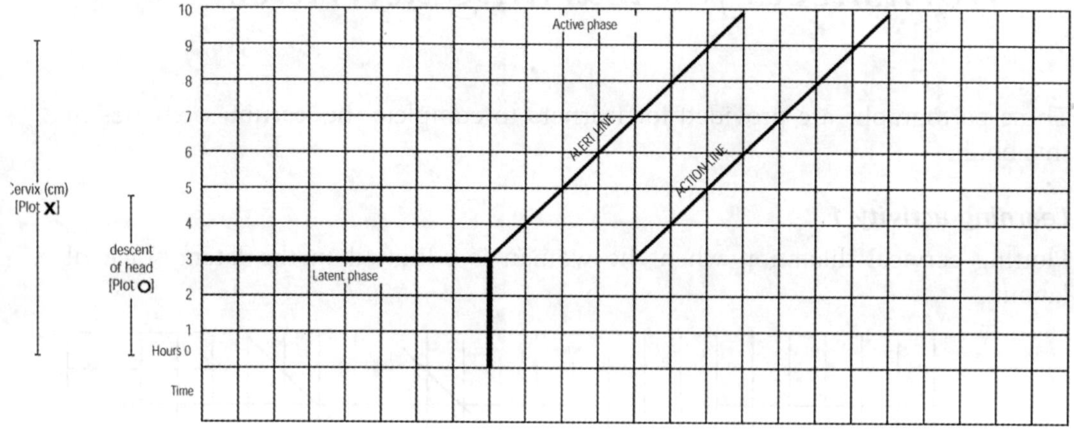

Learning activity 4

Plotting engagement of the fetal head

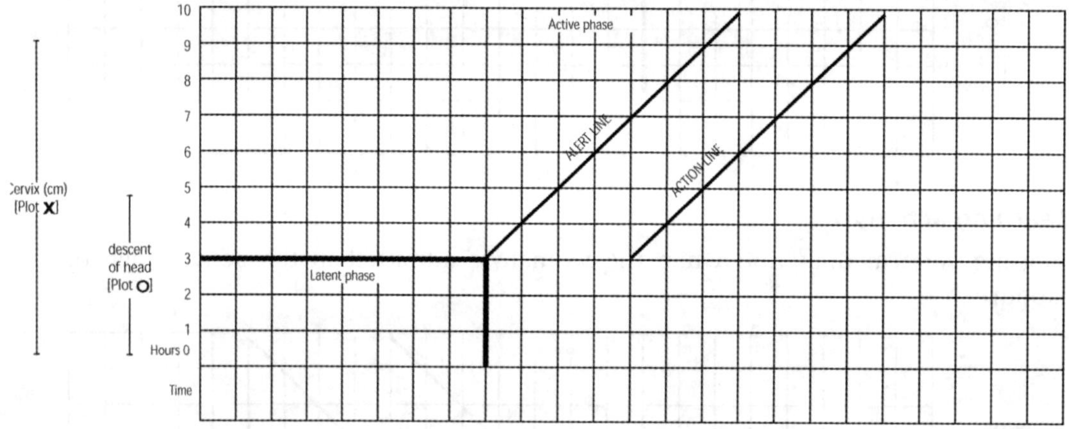

Learning activity 5

Plotting uterine contractions

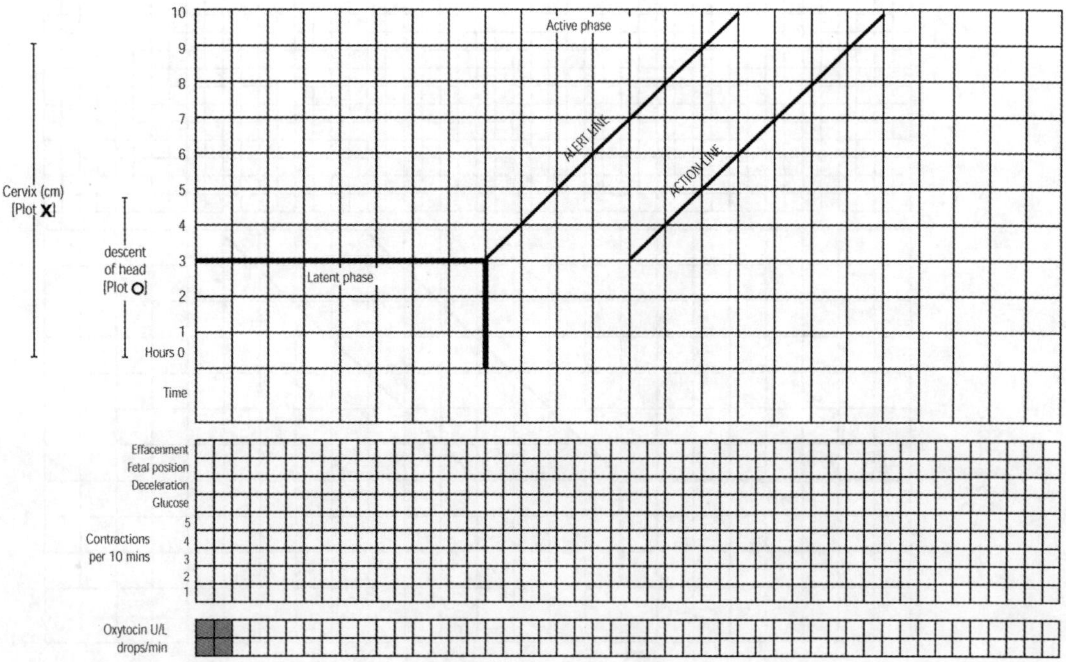

Learning activity 6

Plotting other vaginal examination information

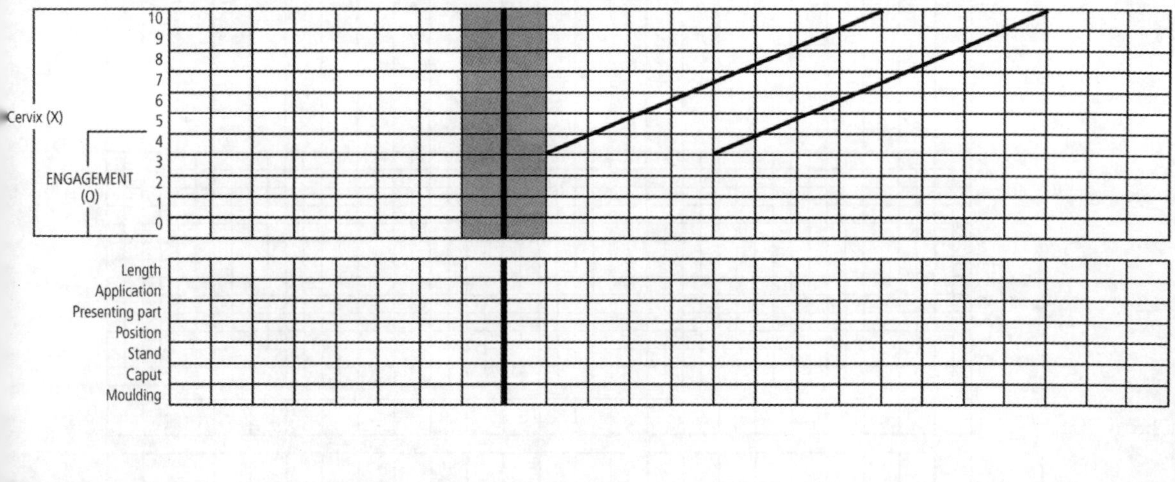

Learning activity 7

Plotting the fetal condition

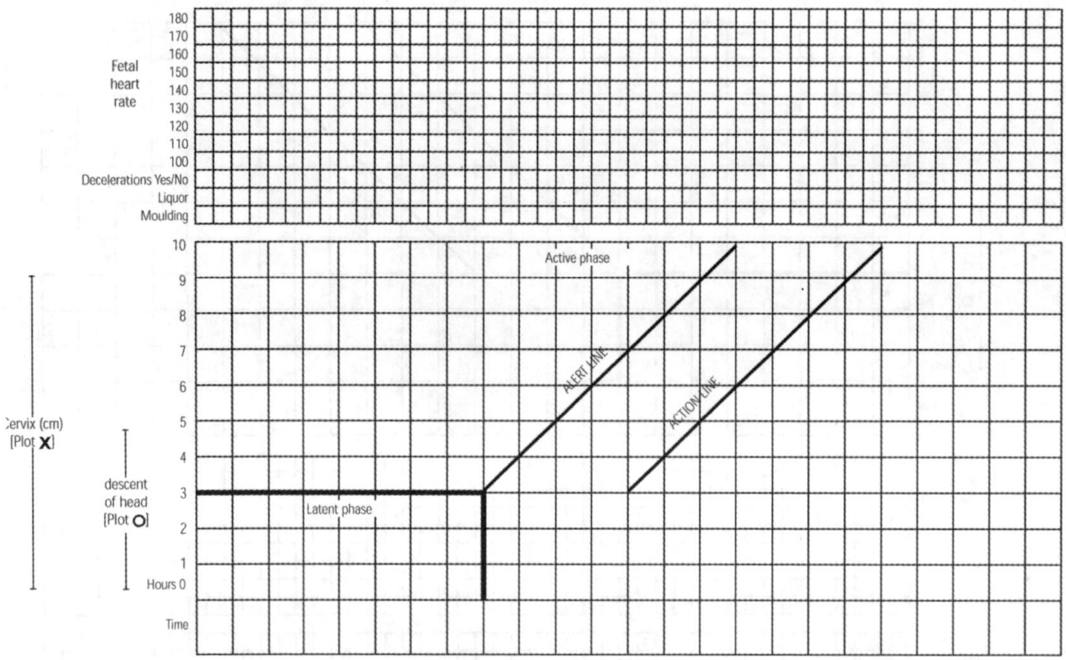

Learning activity 8

Plotting the maternal condition

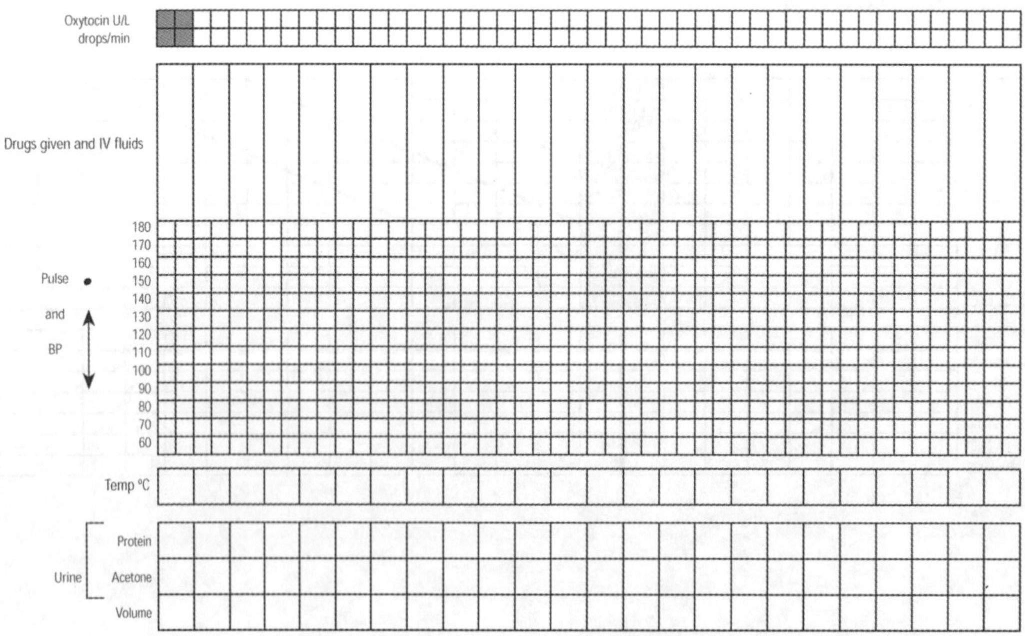

Learning activity 9

A completed partograph

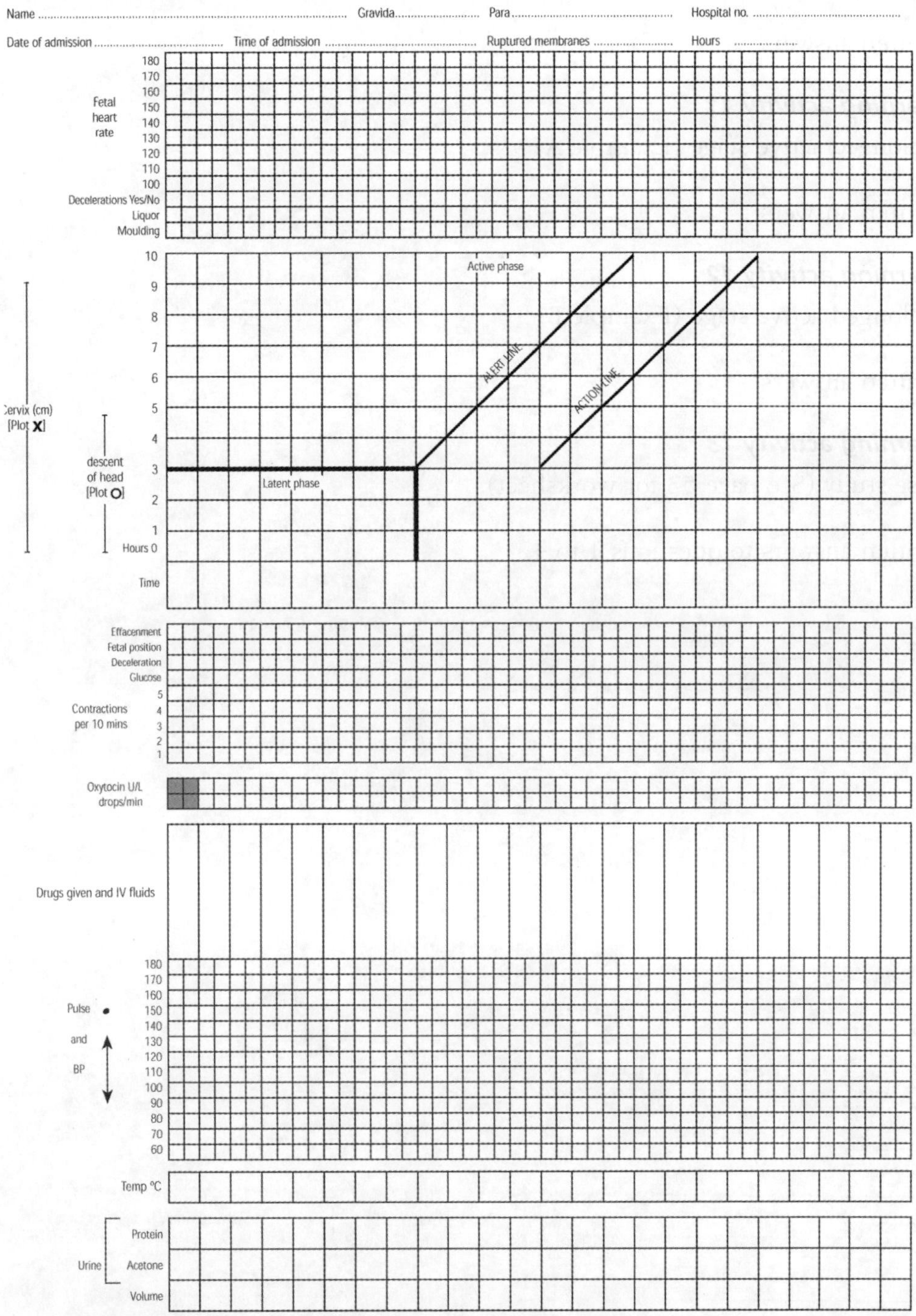

Learning activity 10

Prolonged latent stage

Written answers.

Learning activity 11

Prolonged active stage (Example A)

Written answers.

Learning activity 12

Prolonged active stage (Example B)

Written answers.

Learning activity 13

Case study (See page 53 for worksheet)

Written answers to questions 1 to 4.

Name .... Gravida.......................... Para.. Hospital no. ....

Date of admission .... Time of admission .... Ruptured membranes .... Hours ....

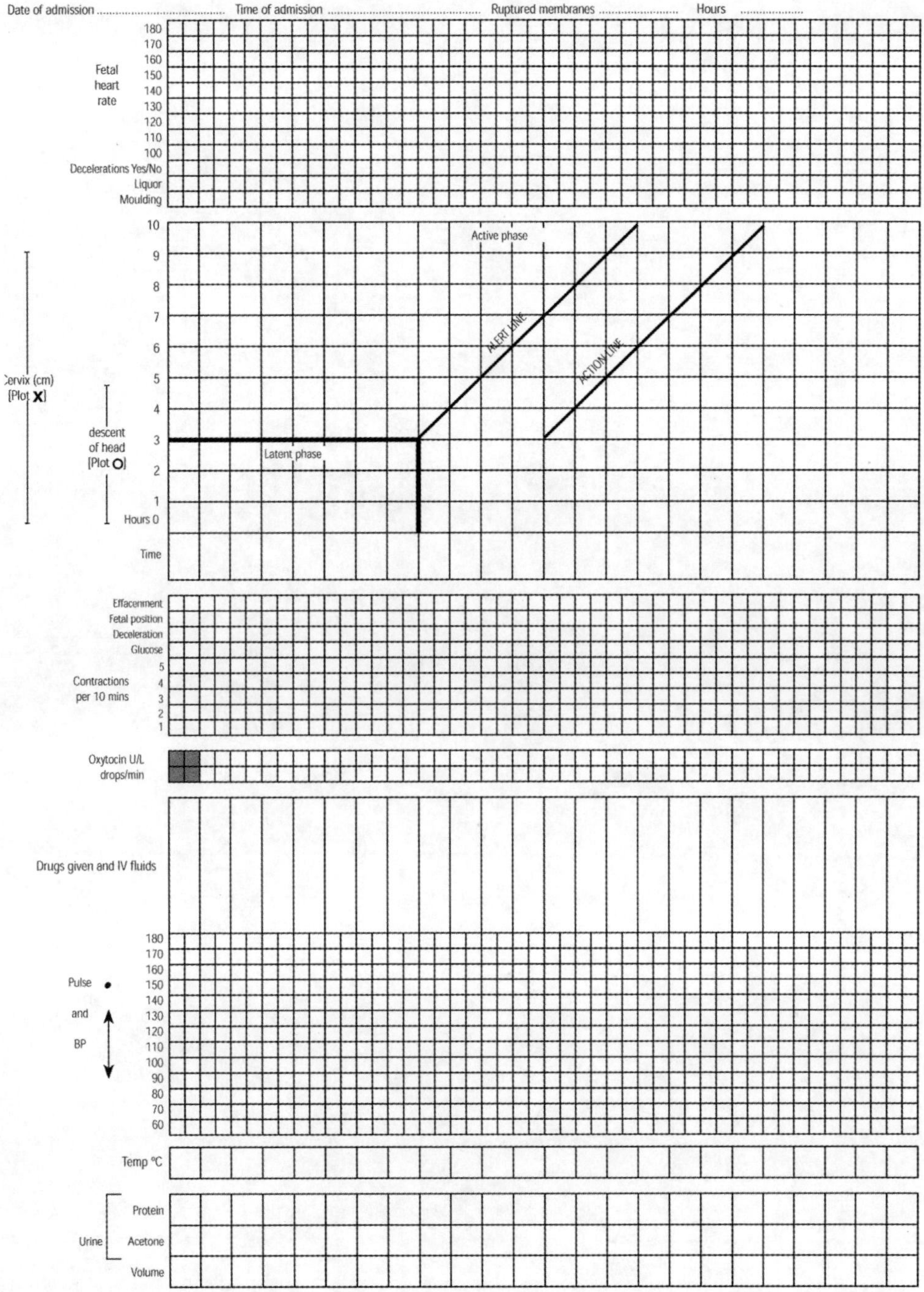

Answers to learning activities

Learning activity 1

Plotting cervical dilatation when a woman is admitted in the latent stage of labour

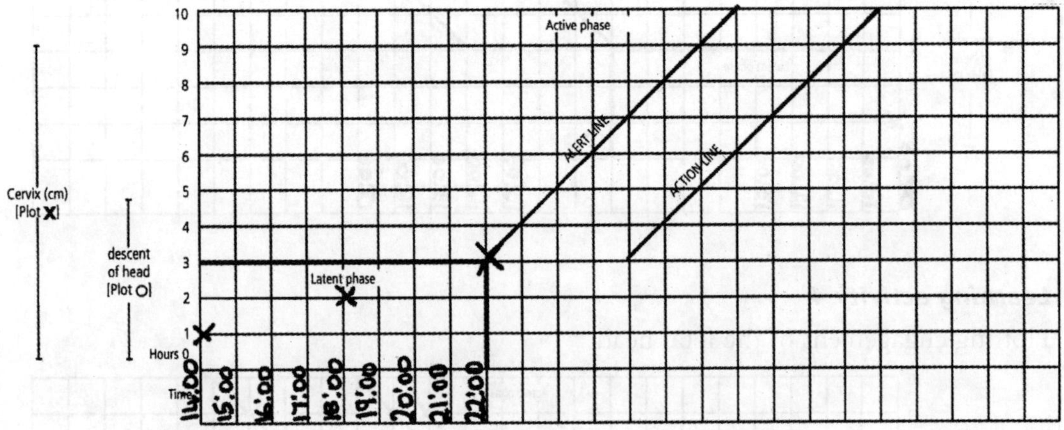

Learning activity 2

Plotting cervical dilatation when a woman is admitted in the active stage of labour

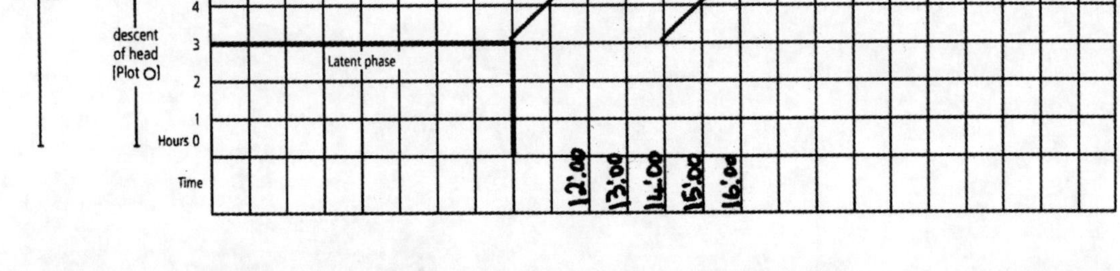

Learning activity 3

Plotting cervical dilatation when a woman is admitted in the latent stage, but proceeds to the active stage before eight hours have elapsed

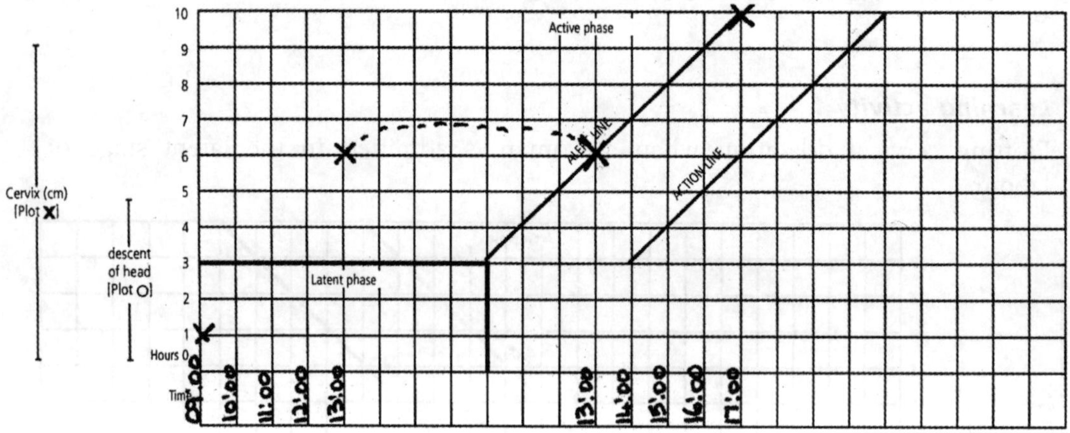

Learning activity 4

Plotting engagement of the fetal head

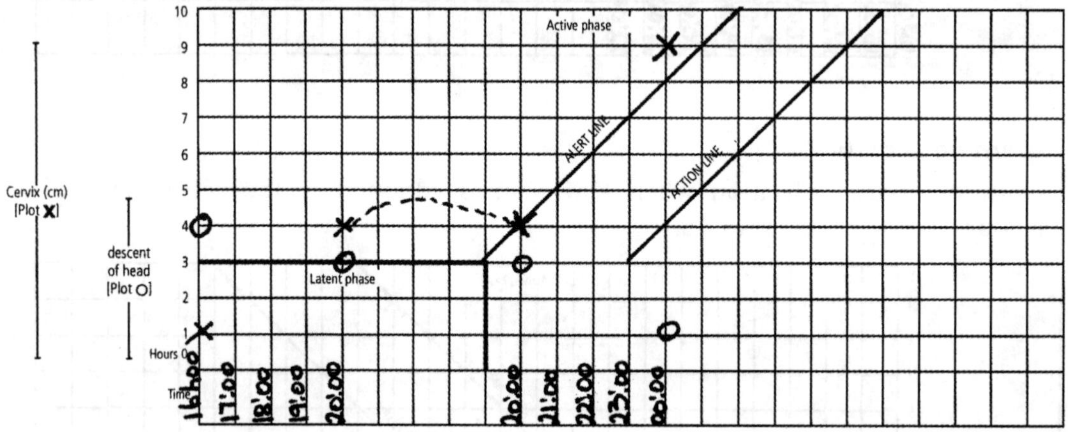

Learning activity 5

Plotting other vaginal examination information

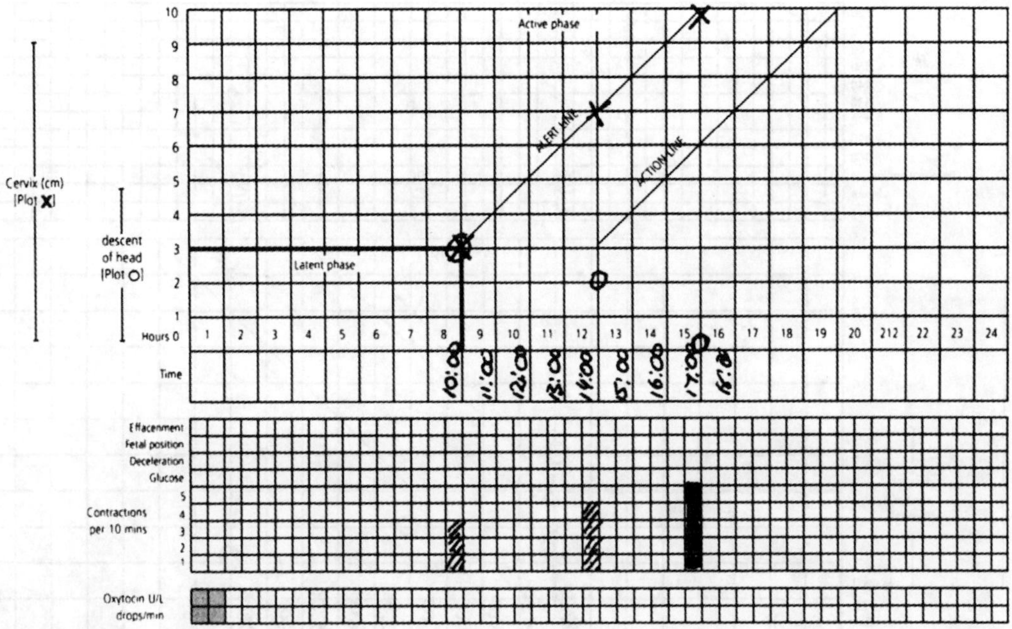

Learning activity 6

Plotting uterine contractions

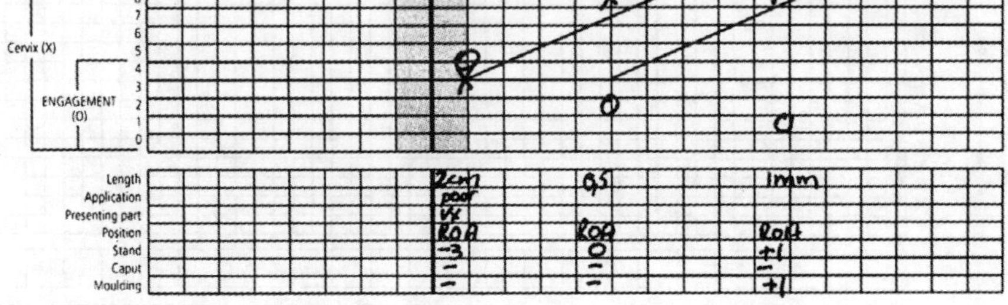

Learning activity 7

Plotting the fetal condition

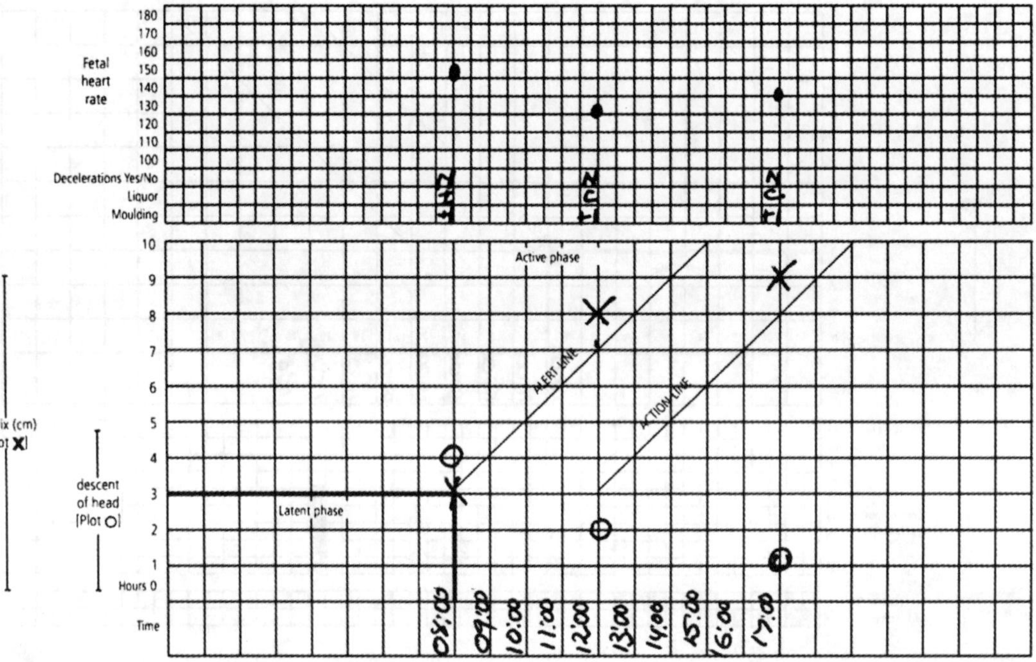

Learning activity 8

Plotting the maternal condition

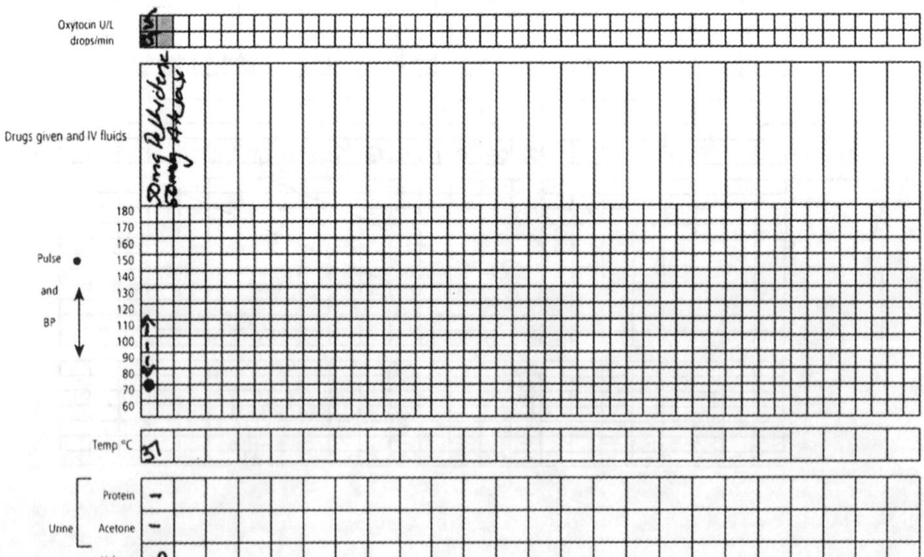

Learning activity 9

A completed partograph

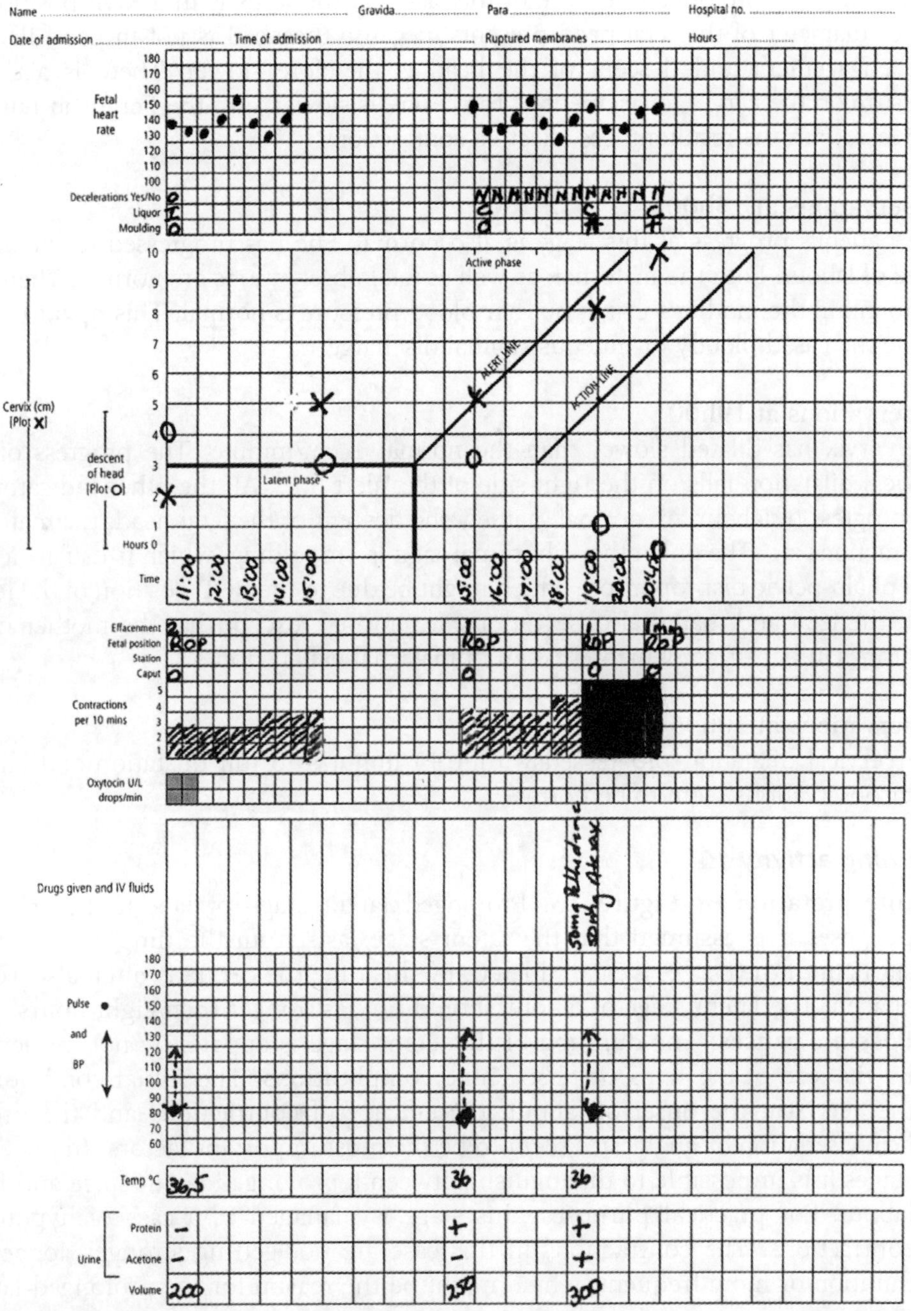

Admission at 11h00

Everything seems to be normal at this stage. The patient is still in the latent phase of labour and both the maternal, as well as fetal observations are in the normal ranges. Labour may be prolonged because of the fact that the fetus is in a ROP position. A bigger diameter of the fetal head presents, because the head is not in good flexion. The engagement and descent of the head is therefore slower. There is also less pressure on the cervix, effacement of the cervix is slower, and the Ferguson reflex is also less, with the resultant less effective contractions.

Observations at 15h00

The patient's progress at this stage is also normal. She has progressed to the active stage of labour. Both the maternal, as well as fetal observations are normal. There is a + protein in the mother's urine, but her blood pressure is normal. This might be due to the increased bloody or mucous vaginal discharge,

Observations at 19h00

The cervix has dilated slower than the normal 1 cm/minute. The progress of the cervical dilatation falls on the right side of the 'alert line'. All the other indicators of the progress of labour are normal, namely the descent of the fetal head, the maternal contractions etc. The only other 'abnormal' sign is +moulding, which is usually a sign of cephalo-pelvic disproportion, which might be due to the ROP position of the fetus. Both the fetal and maternal observations are normal, except that the mother has a + ketones in her urine, which is a sign of maternal exhaustion.

Observations at 20h45

The cervical dilatation progressed within 45 minutes to full dilatation and all the orher observations seem to be normal

Learning activity 10

1. **Interpretation of Figure 13**: Prolonged latent stage of labour. For clinical purposes it is assumed that the latent stage lasts from the time when labour starts until the cervix is 3 cm dilated. By this time the cervix is often also 100% effaced. The latent stage of labour should not last longer than eight hours.
2. **Possible causes**: The duration of the latent stage is apparently not influenced by the size of the fetus or obstructive complications. The initial condition of the cervix at the onset of labour, the efficacy of contractions and the use of heavy sedation or analgesics seem to be the most important factors. In the early stages it is impossible to distinguish between a prolonged latent stage and false labour. For practical purposes, this stage is managed as a case of hypotonic contractions. The contractions in this case are not getting stronger, longer in duration or more frequent, which might be the reason for the prolonged latent stage in this case.

3. **Management of problems**: In the latent stage it is difficult to distinguish between primary hypotonic inertia and what is known as false labour. If the membranes have ruptured, labour must be stimulated with oxytocin. If they are intact, the easiest way to manage the problem is by sedating the patient and, if necessary, to give an analgesic such as Pethidine, so that the patient can rest and sleep. When the patient awakes, she is likely to be in active labour (85%) or contractions will have disappeared completely (10%). In the first case, labour is then managed according to normal routine. In the latter case a diagnosis of false labour can be made and the patient may be transferred to the antenatal ward or be discharged. This could possibly have been done at 13:00.

The aim is to save the patient the unnecessary pain and exhaustion of ineffective uterine function and is often also of a diagnostic nature.

If the inertia continues, the contractions must be stimulated with oxytocin (augmentation of labour). The membranes should be kept intact as long as possible.

Augmentation of labour according to *Guidelines for Maternity Care in South Africa* (2002)

1. Add two units of oxytocin to 1 litre of Ringer's lactate.
2. Start infusion at a rate of 15 drops per minute (d.p.m.) (60 ml/per hour).
3. Increase the rate by 15 d.p.m. every 30 minutes until a minimum of three strong contractions in 10 minutes are achieved.
4. The infusion rate should not exceed 60 d.p.m.

Learning activity 11

1. **Interpretation of Figure 14**: The active stage of labour is prolonged, possibly because of cephalopelvic disproportion (CDP) caused by the posterior position of the fetal occiput. Signs of CPD are present (moulding and high fetal head) at 10:00. The patient should have been referred to a hospital (in the case of a clinic), or the doctor should have been called. Ketoacidosis is also present, which might have an influence later on the effectivity of the contractions, and might lead to fetal distress. The fetal and maternal conditions seem to be normal.
2. **Possible causes: Assessment of four Ps**
   - *Abnormality of uterine contractions (Powers):* The contractions seem to be normal.
   - *Abnormalities of the fetus (Passenger):*
     Abnormalities of position, namely the **occipito-posterior position**, can cause a prolonged first and second stage of labour for the following reasons:
     - Cephalopelvic disproportion (CPD): This is quite common because an abnormal diameter of the fetus has to pass through the birth canal.

- Abnormal uterine muscle function: The contractions are often hypotonic and uncoordinated, possibly because the presenting part is not well applied to cervix.
- Dilatation of the cervix: This is retarded and often incomplete, owing to abnormal uterine muscle function as well as poor application of the presenting part.
- The presenting part: The presenting part remains high.
- Membranes: Membranes often rupture very early in labour with the resulting danger of intra-uterine infection.

- *Abnormalities of the birth canal (Passage):*
  See above. There seems to be cephalopelvic disproportion (CPD). Moulding has been ++ since 10:00.
- *Abnormalities relating to the woman (Patient):*
  Certain factors relating to the patient may contribute to prolonged labour:
  - Maternal exhaustion and ketoacidosis are a common result of prolonged labour, owing to the increased uterine work that is necessary. Poor management, for example, insufficient sedation or calorie intake, may aggravate the condition. This mother experienced ketoacidosis at 14:00.
  - Women experience more discomfort and pain in prolonged labour because of the pressure that the occiput area of the fetus exerts on the maternal sacrum. Excessive pain leads to fear, which may aggravate pain. The result is secretion of catecholamines, which cause irregular and ineffective uterine contractions. As a result of the pain and fear, a woman may also contract her pelvic floor muscles, which will prevent engagement and descent.

3. **Management of the condition:**
   a) The head is too high to rupture the membranes; prolapse of the cord is a possibility. In addition, mother-to-child transmission of HIV is a bigger possibility with ruptured membranes.
   b) The caregiver should evaluate quality of contractions carefully. Augmentation should not be considered after 10:00 because signs of CPD are present (moulding and high fetal head).
   c) An IV infusion is always a good choice in the case of prolonged labour, because of the possibility of postpartum haemorrhage and the possibility of interventions. There are + ketones in the patient's urine, so it might be a good idea to use a half dextrose and saline solution or a Ringer's lactate infusion. It seems fairly certain that this mother will go for a caesarean section, and she should therefore be kept nil per os after 10:00.
   d) The woman should be encouraged to remain mobile for as long as possible during the first stage of labour, as walking increases her level of comfort and promotes less frequent, more efficient contractions. It also encourages

engagement and descent of the presenting part, while serving to distract her attention from the discomfort of her contractions.

When backache occurs because of the posterior position of the occiput, changes in position can facilitate rotation and promote maternal comfort and relaxation. An all-fours or side-lying position, combined with the pelvic rocking motion, may be used to turn an occipito-posterior fetus to a more favorable position. Another position that may help with rotation of an occipito-posterior position is the lunge. It widens the side of the pelvis towards which the mother is lunging. When the mother became tired (probably after 10:00) – she should have been nursed in a side-lying position.

e) Non-pharmacological pain relief methods may bring some relief, but the labour is too far advanced to start with it now. The contractions are very strong after 10:00 and the mother may experience much pain then. An analgesic, for example, Pethidine, in the usual dose of 50 to 100 mg and Aterax 50 mg intramuscularly, can be administered if the patient cannot bear the pain anymore.

f) The patient should be referred to a hospital!

Learning activity 12

1. To answer this question, you need to interpret Figure 15 on page 40 and assess the four Ps:
   - *Abnormality of uterine contractions (Powers):* The contractions are not strong enough and the duration is not long enough.
   - *Abnormalities of the fetus (Passenger):* There seem to be no abnormalities of the fetus – it is in an occipito-anterior position. There are signs of fetal distress as indicated by the late decelerations since 16:00.
   - *Abnormalities of the birth canal (Passage):* Abnormalities of the bony pelvis, for example, of the pelvic inlet, mid-pelvis and pelvic outlet, may cause prolonged labour. There are no clear signs of CPD here. Engagement of the fetal head is slow, but there is no moulding.
   - *Abnormalities of the woman (Patient):* There are no signs of maternal distress or other abnormalities. The contractions are not very strong. The maternal reaction to pain should be observed.

   Conclusion: It seems as if ineffective contractions might be the reason for the prolonged labour.
2. **Management of the condition**

   a) The head is too high to rupture membranes. Prolapse of the cord is a possibility. In addition, mother-to-child transmission of HIV is also a bigger possibility with ruptured membranes. However, it may stimulate the uterus to contract better if the head fits better on the cervix. The membranes can be ruptured carefully if the patient is in a hospital. The fetal heart rate should be observed carefully for signs of prolapse of the cord.

b) Before augmenting labour, evaluate the quality of contractions carefully. Augmentation at 14:00 might help. There are no signs of CPD, and better contractions might help the fetus get through the pelvis (also see the augmentation regime on page 33). An oxytocin infusion must be stopped immediately if:
   - hypertonic uterine contractions occur, or
   - the pattern of the fetal heart beat becomes abnormal.

c) Adequate maternal hydration and nutrition: An IV infusion is always a good choice in the case of prolonged labour (see Learning activity 11, question 3(c).) There are no ketones in the patient's urine, so Ringer's lactate might be a good choice for the IV infusion. The woman can suck on hard sweets, or drink sweet cooldrinks or fruit juice. This provides in her energy and her fluid needs. A practice that patients have found acceptable is to wrap a piece of ice in gauze for them to suck. This enables the woman to keep her lips and throat moist without the danger of inadvertent aspiration of ice or large gulps of water.

d) The woman should be encouraged to remain mobile for as long as possible during the first stage of labour, as walking will increase her level of comfort and promote less frequent, more efficient contractions. It also encourages engagement and descent of the presenting part, while serving to distract her attention from the discomfort of her contractions (see Learning activity 11).

e) Non-pharmacological pain relief methods may bring some relief. Pethidine and Aterax can be given if the patient cannot bear the pain anymore. The contractions do not seem to be too strong.

Learning activity 13

1. a) See the completed partograph on page 65.

   b) The patient is a primigravida with a normal pregnancy and she is in the latent stage of labour. Maternal observations seem to be normal. The fetal observations are normal too. As far as the four Ps are concerned:
   - The contractions seem to be normal for this stage of labour.
   - The fetal head is in a normal anterior position.
   - The fact that the head is still 3/5 above the pubis is a possible problem. The fetal head usually starts to engage at 36 weeks of pregnancy in the case of a primigravida and should be 4/5 in the pelvis at 40 weeks of pregnancy. The 'high' head can be the result of placenta praevia or cephalopelvic disproportion (CPD). The application of the fetal presenting part on the cervix is also poor.
   - The mother is tense and anxious.

   Conclusion: Benilo is a 'normal' primipara in the latent stage of labour. Progress of labour should be monitored very carefully to exclude the possibility of CPD or placenta praevia.

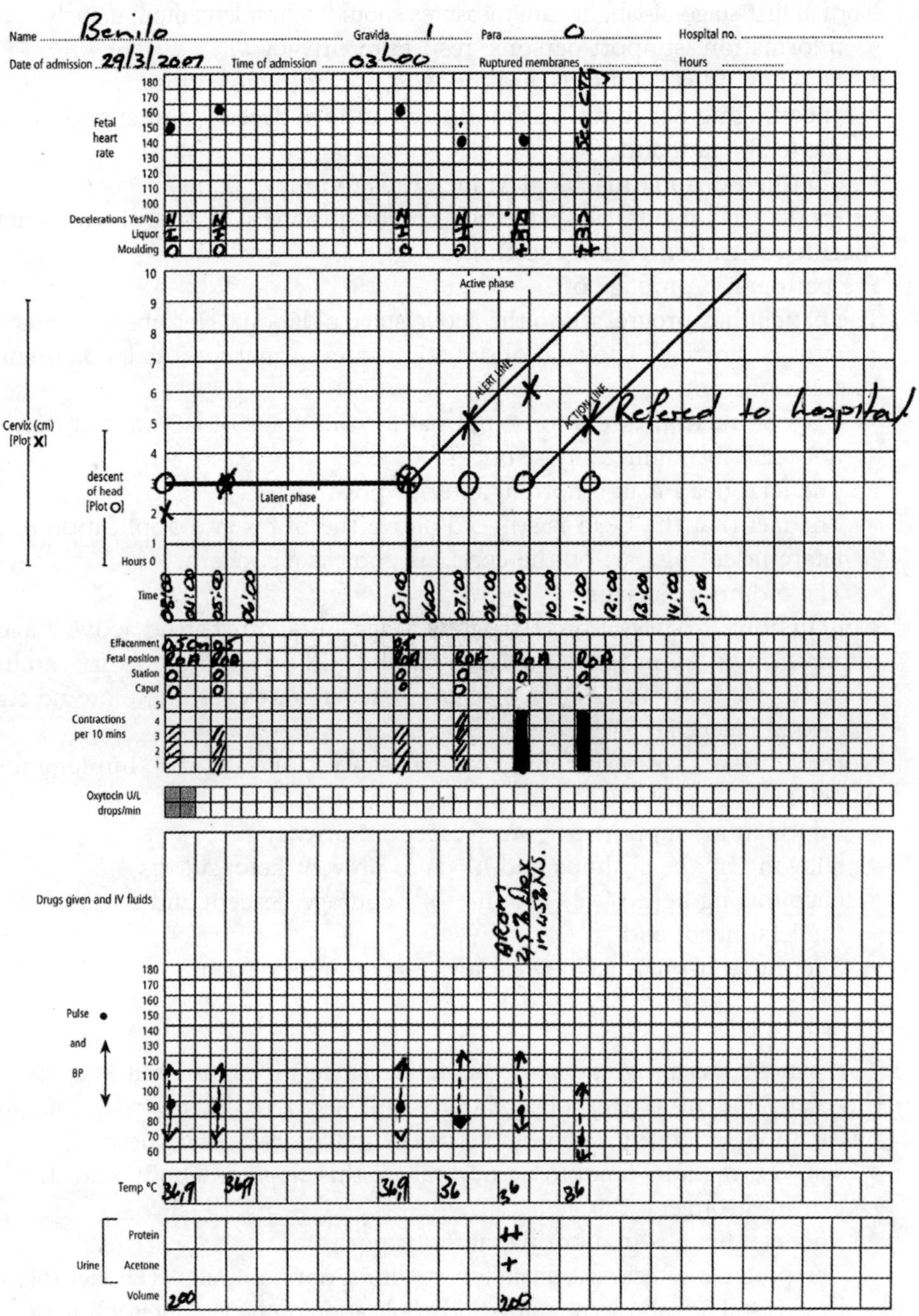

Name Benilo
Gravida 1
Para 0
Hospital no.
Date of admission 29/3/2007
Time of admission 03h00
Ruptured membranes
Hours
Fetal heart rate
Decelerations Yes/No
Liquor
Moulding
Active phase
ALERT LINE
ACTION LINE
Refered to hospital
Cervix (cm) [Plot X]
descent of head [Plot O]
Latent phase
Hours
Time
Effacement
Fetal position
Station
Caput
Contractions per 10 mins
Oxytocin U/L drops/min
Drugs given and IV fluids
Pulse ●
and
BP
Temp °C
Urine
Protein
Acetone
Volume

c) Normal first-stage-of-labour care measures should be implemented, namely:
   - information, support persons, respect of privacy,
   - allowing intake of fluids and foods to prevent ketoacidosis,
   - encouraging her to walk around to encourage descent and engagement of the fetal head, and
   - offering non-pharmacological measures to relieve pain.

   Referral to a hospital will depend on the progress of labour and on the specific referral criteria of the clinic.

2. a) See partograph on page 65.
   b) The patient has progressed to the active stage of labour. Her observations still seem to be normal. The fetal observations are normal too. As far as the four Ps are concerned:
   - The contractions seem to be normal for this stage of labour, but they are not really becoming any stronger.
   - The fetal head is in a normal anterior position.
   - The fact that the head is still 3/5 above the pubis and application of the fetal presenting part on the cervix is poor, is a concern.
   - The mother is in pain.

   Conclusion: Progress from the latent stage of labour to the active stage is normal. However, progress of labour should still be monitored very carefully to exclude a possible CPD or placenta praevia. However, there are no signs of vaginal bleeding.
   c) Normal first-stage-of-labour care measures should be implemented, namely:
   - information, support persons, respect of privacy,
   - allowing intake of fluids and foods to prevent ketoacidosis,
   - encouraging her to walk around to encourage descent and engagement of the fetal head, and
   - offering non-pharmacological measures to relieve pain.

3. a) See partograph on page 65.
   b) The patient has progressed to the active stage of labour, but she falls on the alert line now. Her observations still seem to be normal. The fetal observations are normal too. As far as the four Ps are concerned:
   - The contractions seem to be normal for this stage of labour, and they are getting stronger.
   - The fetal head is in a normal anterior position.
   - The progress of cervical dilatation is within normal limits. The fact that the head is still 3/5 above the pubis and application of the fetal presenting part on the cervix is poor, is worrying. The progress of engagement of the fetal head should be observed carefully as the contractions are becoming stronger.
   - The mother is in pain.

Conclusion: Progress of cervical dilatation in the active stage is normal, but progress of engagement and descent of the fetal head is not. No signs of moulding or caput are present at the moment. Progress of labour should still be monitored very carefully to exclude a possible CPD. The mother has not emptied her bladder since 03:00 and should be encouraged to do so to prevent a full bladder from obstructing progress of labour.

Normal first-stage-of-labour care measures should still be implemented, namely:

- information, support persons, respect of privacy,
- allowing intake of fluids and foods to prevent ketoacidosis,
- encouraging her to walk around to encourage descent and engagement of the fetal head, and
- offering non-pharmacological measures for pain relief, depending on the practical guidelines of the clinic and the regulations of the South African Nursing Council (SANC).

4. **Observations of partograph at 09:00 (see figure on page 65):**

(a) The patient has not progressed normally in the active stage of labour. Her cervical dilatation was slower than it should have been and fell on the right of the alert line at 09:00. There was no progress in the engagement of the fetal head. The maternal observations still seemed to be normal, but she developed ketoacidosis at 09:00. The membranes were ruptured artificially and there was meconium in the liquor. The fetal observations seemed normal. As far as the four Ps are concerned:

- The contractions seemed normal for this stage of labour, and they were getting stronger.
- The fetal head was in a normal anterior position.
- The progress of the cervical dilatation was **not** within normal limits anymore. The fact that the head was still 3/5 above the pubis and application of the fetal presenting part on the cervix was poor, is worrying. In addition, moulding and caput have developed. There was no progress either in effacement or application of the cervix.

Conclusion: Progress of cervical dilatation in the active stage is abnormal, as well as engagement and descent of the fetal head. Signs of moulding and caput are present. The ketoacidosis of the mother should be reversed as soon as possible, or it will have a negative effect on the effectivity of the contractions and the well-being of the fetus. It is not clear why the membranes were ruptured. Perhaps this was done to see whether this would help the fetal head engage. The rupturing of membranes was a dangerous decision, as the fetal head is high and there is a possibility of prolapse of the cord. **The patient should have been referred to a hospital immediately!**

5. **Observations of partograph at 11:00 (see figure on page 65):**
   a) There are now signs of fetal distress as well as clear signs of CPD. **THE PATIENT SHOULD HAVE BEEN REFERRED TO A HOSPITAL IMMEDIATELY!**
   b) CPD is the main reason for prolonged labour in this case.
   c) The day staff should have realised that the patient should be referred to a hospital around 9:00 that morning! Instead, they allowed labour to continue until the night staff came on duty a full ten hours later, by which time various complications had set in as a result of CPD.

Bibliography

Crichton, D. 1974. Better clinical diagnosis of contraction of the transverse brim. *South African Medical Journal* 48: 781.

Cronjé, H. S. and Grobler, C. J. F. 2003. *Obstetrics in Southern Africa*. 2nd edition. Pretoria: Van Schaik.

De Kock, J. and Van der Walt, C. 2004. *Maternal and Newborn Care: A Complete Guide for Midwives and other Health Professionals.* Pretoria: Juta.

Department of Health. 2002. *Guidelines for Maternity Care in South Africa. A Manual for Clinics, Community Health Centres and District Hospitals.* Pretoria: Department of Health.

Department of Health. 2006. *Third Report on Confidential Enquiries into Maternal Deaths in South Africa 2002–2004*. Pretoria: Department of Health.

Enkin, M., Keirse, M. J. N. C., Neilson, J., Crowther, C., Hodnett, E. and Hofmeyr, J. 2000. *A Guide to Effective Care in Pregnancy and Childbirth.* 3rd edition. Oxford: Oxford University Press.

Fahdhy, M. and Chongsuvivatwong, C. 2005. Evaluation of World Health Organization Partograph Implementation by Midwives for Maternity Home Birth in Medan, Indonesia. *Midwifery* 21(4): 301–310.

Lavender, T., Alfirevic, Z. and Walkinshaw, S. 1998. Partograph action line study: A randomized trial. *British Journal of Obstetrics and Gynaecology*. Sept 105(9): 976-980.

Lavender, T., Alfirevic, Z. and Walkinshaw, S. 2006. Effect of different partograph action lines on birth outcomes: A randomized controlled trial. *Obstetrics and Gynaecology.* Aug 108(2): 295–302.

Nolte, A. G. W. (Ed.) 1998. *A Textbook for Midwives.* Pretoria: Van Schaik.

Odberg Petterson, K., Svensson, M.-L. and Christensson, K. 2000. Evaluation of an adapted model of the World Health Organization partograph used by Angolan midwives in a peripheral delivery unit. *Midwifery* 16(2): 82–88.

Perinatal Education Programme. *Maternal Care Manual 1.* Cape Town: Periodical Education Trust.

World Health Organization. 1994. *Preventing Prolonged Labour: A Practical Guide. Part I – IV.* Geneva: Maternal Health and Safe Motherhood Programme – Division of Family Health.

World Health Organization. 1996. *Obstructed Labour Module.* Geneva: Maternal Health and Safe Motherhood Programme – Division of Family Health.

Index